CLINICAL CASES IN ENDOCRINOLOGY

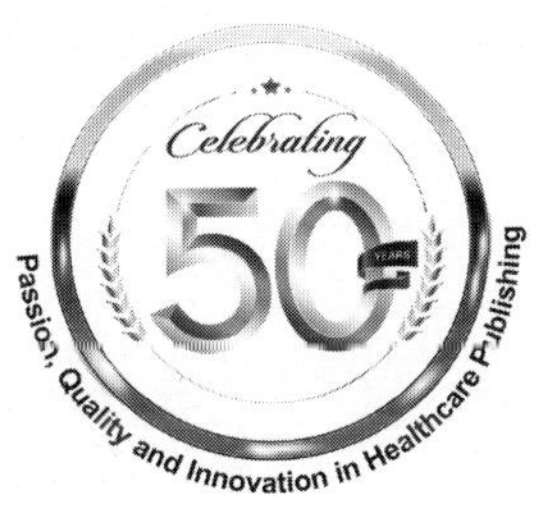

CLINICAL CASES IN ENDOCRINOLOGY

Editor

Pramila Kalra

MD DM (Endocrinology) MNAMS FACE (USA)

Professor

Department of Endocrinology and Metabolism

Ramaiah Medical College

Bengaluru, Karnataka, India

Foreword

Prasanna Kumar KM

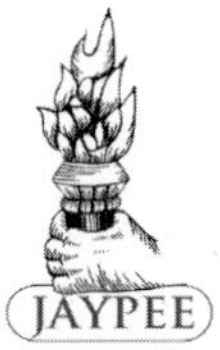

JAYPEE BROTHERS MEDICAL PUBLISHERS

The Health Sciences Publisher

New Delhi | London | Panama

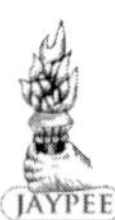

Jaypee Brothers Medical Publishers (P) Ltd.

Headquarters
Jaypee Brothers Medical Publishers (P) Ltd
4838/24, Ansari Road, Daryaganj
New Delhi 110 002, India
Phone: +91-11-43574357
Fax: +91-11-43574314
Email: jaypee@jaypeebrothers.com

Overseas Offices
J.P. Medical Ltd
83 Victoria Street, London
SW1H 0HW (UK)
Phone: +44 20 3170 8910
Fax: +44 (0)20 3008 6180
Email: info@jpmedpub.com

Jaypee-Highlights Medical Publishers Inc
City of Knowledge, Bld. 235, 2nd Floor
Clayton, Panama City, Panama
Phone: +1 507-301-0496
Fax: +1 507-301-0499
Email: cservice@jphmedical.com

Jaypee Brothers Medical Publishers (P) Ltd
Bhotahity, Kathmandu, Nepal
Phone: +977-9741283608
Email: kathmandu@jaypeebrothers.com

Website: www.jaypeebrothers.com
Website: www.jaypeedigital.com

Inquiries for bulk sales may be solicited at: jaypee@jaypeebrothers.com

Clinical Cases in Endocrinology

First Edition: **2019**

ISBN: 978-93-5270-589-4

Printed at Rajkamal Electric Press, Kundli, Haryana.

Dedicated to

My parents for their support throughout my career
To my teachers who made me capable of reaching this level
To my husband and my daughter for their constant moral support
To my brother for his moral support
To my patients and individuals who have endocrine problems in the hope that this book will help to alleviate their sufferings by spreading some knowledge in the field

Contributors

Altamash Shaikh
MD (Medicine) DNB (Endocrinology)
Consultant Endocrinologist
Saifee Hospital
Mumbai, Maharashtra, India

Anu Vishwanath
MBBS DAB (Pediatric Endocrinology)
Consultant Endocrinologist
Children's Hospital of Illinois
OSF Saint Francis Medical Center
Peoria, Illinois, USA

BS Narendra
MD (Medicine) DM (Endocrinology)
Consultant Endocrinologist
Apollo Hospitals
Bengaluru, Karnataka, India

Chitra S
MD (Medicine) DM (Endocrinology) MRCUP (UK) Endocrinology (SCE)
Assistant Professor
Department of Endocrinology
Ramaiah Memorial Hospital
Bengaluru, Karnataka, India

Dinesh Kumar Singh
MBBS
Junior Resident (Medicine)
Endocrinology Unit
Department of Medicine
King George's Medical University
Lucknow, Uttar Pradesh, India

KVS Harikumar
MD (Medicine) DM (Endocrinology)
Consultant Endocrinologist
Assistant Professor
Department of Medicine and Endocrinology
Command Hospital
Chandigarh, India

Madhukar Mittal
MD (Medicine) DM (Endocrinology)
Head
Department of Medical Endocrinology
King George's Medical University
Lucknow, Uttar Pradesh, India

Manzer AS
MD
Consultant Fertility Specialist
(Obstetrician and Gynecologist)
Saifee Hospital
Mumbai, Maharashtra, India

Neelam Yadav
MBBS
Junior Resident
Endocrinology Unit
Department of Medicine
King George's Medical University
Lucknow, Uttar Pradesh, India

Neeraj Garg
MD DM (Endocrinology)
Associate Consultant
SPS Hospitals
Ludhiana, Punjab, India

Pradyut Tiwari
MBBS
Junior Resident
Department of Medicine
King George's Medical University
Lucknow, Uttar Pradesh, India

Pramila Kalra
MD DM (Endocrinology) MNAMS FACE (USA)
Professor
Department of Endocrinology and Metabolism
Ramaiah Medical College
Bengaluru, Karnataka, India

Prashant Kaduskar
MD DM (Endocrinology)
Consultant Endocrinologist
Columbia Asia Hospital
Pune, Maharashtra, India

Rajeshwari Janakiraman
MD DM (Endocrinology)
Consultant
Columbia Asia Referral Hospital-Yeshwanthpur
Bengaluru, Karnataka, India

Sambit Das
MD DM (Endocrinology)
Consultant Endocrinologist
Bhubaneshwar, Odisha, India

Satyendra Sonkar
MD (Medicine)
Associate Professor
Department of Medicine
King George's Medical University
Lucknow, Uttar Pradesh, India

Shobhith Shakya
MBBS
Junior Resident
Endocrinology Unit
Department of Medicine
King George's Medical University
Lucknow, Uttar Pradesh, India

Sunil Kota
MD (Medicine) DM (Endocrinology)
Consultant Endocrinologist
CARE Hospitals
Hyderabad, Telangana, India

V Sri Nagesh
MD (Medicine) DM (Endocrinology)
Consultant Endocrinologist
Endocare Hospital
Vijayawada, Andhra Pradesh, India

Foreword

The book *Clinical Cases in Endocrinology* edited by Professor Pramila Kalra is a laudable initiative. The book has a clinical approach which makes it very easy for practicing clinicians to understand and appreciate the intricacies of diagnosis and management of complex endocrine diseases. A unique feature of the book is that, the authors across the country, who are young, enthusiastic and have an evidence-based approach to endocrinology. The approach and investigation and discussion of the cases are highly relevant to our country taking into view the infrastructure and the accessibility for these investigations. The frequently ask questions (FAQs) in each case is pragmatic and simple.

Overall the *Clinical Cases in Endocrinology* is a fresh and scientific approach to endocrine cases as endocrinology should be practiced. The book will be of great help to postgraduates and medical students interested in endocrinology to learn the skills of management of endocrine cases. I hope physicians will make use of the knowledge and experience imbibed in this book by the authors, to improve their skills in the management of endocrine cases in future.

Prasanna Kumar KM
Former Senior Professor and Head
Department of Endocrinology
Diabetes and Metabolism
Ramaiah Medical College
Former President
Endocrine Society of India (ESI) and
Research Society of Study of Diabetes in India (RSSDI)

Foreword

Preface

The thought of the book came into my mind about a year back. The typical problem which Endocrinology trainees and broader specialty residents face in India is that they do not have a book in Endocrinology which discusses clinical cases in the real world in a very simple fashion so I thought a case-based approach written in a very straightforward manner would benefit the readers.

The book has been coauthored by many leading Endocrinologists in the field. The book has been written with the daily clinical Endocrinology problems in mind and how the thought process should go further in evaluating these cases.

I have tried to cover most of the important topics in the field of Endocrinology. I hope the book will help residents and upcoming Endocrinology trainees.

Pramila Kalra

Contents

Plate 1

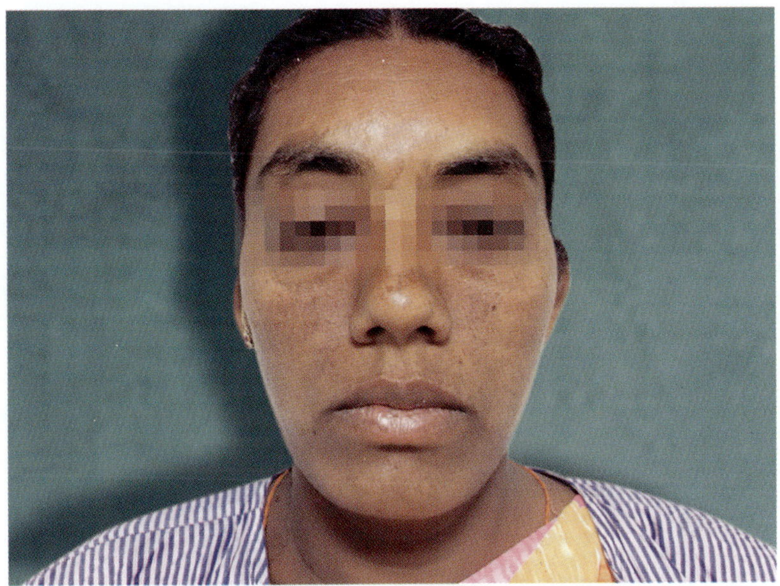

FIG. 1.1 Acromegaly—typical facial features

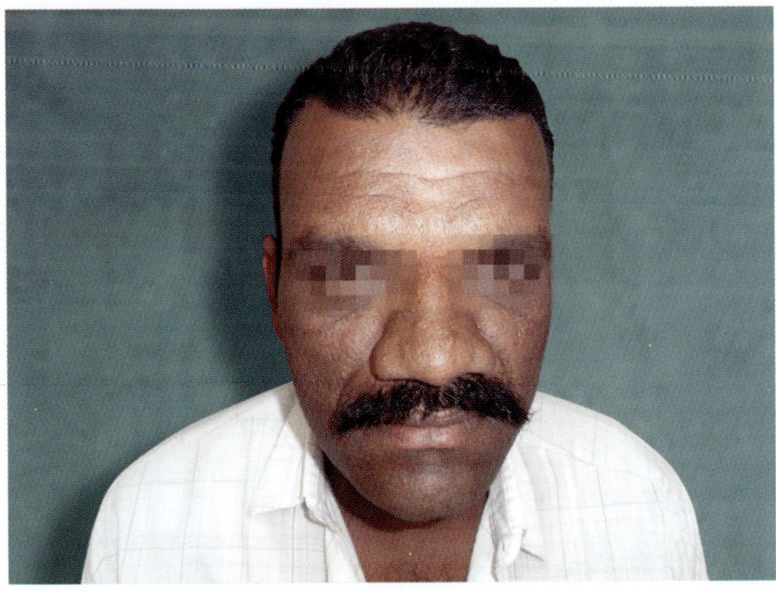

FIG. 1.2 Typical features of acromegaly in a male

Plate 2

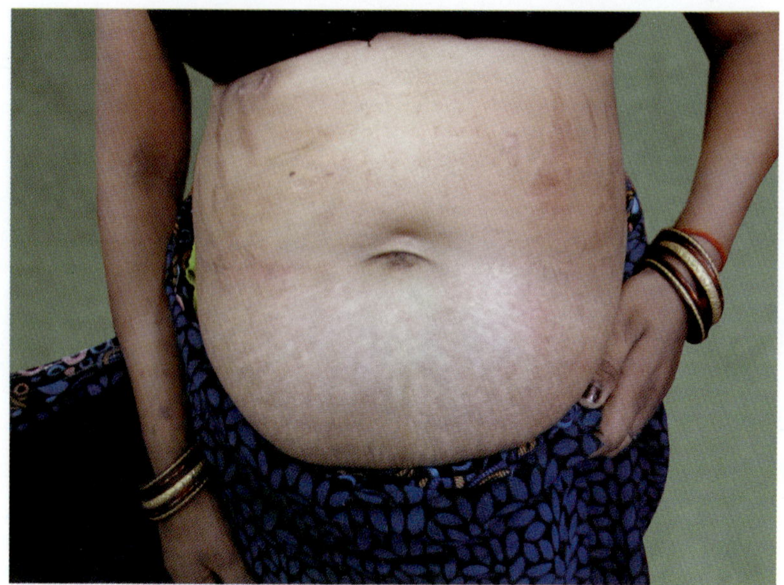

FIG. 2.1 Striae of Cushing's syndrome

CHAPTER

1

Approach to Acromegaly

Pramila Kalra

CASE 1

A 45-year-old lady presents with complaints of a progressive increase in the size of hands and feet and shoe size for past 5 years. The family members have noticed a change in her facial appearance in the form of coarsening of features and her voice has become sonorous. She also has complaints of frequent headaches for past 1 year.

She complains of amenorrhea for past 5 years.

She also has complaints of joint pains for past 3 years which have become more severe for the past 3 months. She is hypertensive for past 1 year and complaints of grade 2 dyspnea on exertion and her hypertension is controlled on 10 mg of cilnidipine and 40 mg of telmisartan. She is not a known diabetic and has checked her random sugars 1 week back which was normal.

She is not on any other medications presently (Fig. 1.1).

Q. 1 When should we suspect acromegaly?

Ans. *The diagnosis of acromegaly is suspected in patients with 2 or more of the following comorbidities:* new-onset diabetes, diffuse arthralgias, new-onset or difficult-to-control hypertension, cardiac disease including biventricular hypertrophy and diastolic or systolic dysfunction, fatigue, headaches, carpal tunnel syndrome, sleep apnea syndrome, diaphoresis, loss of vision, colon polyps, and progressive jaw malocclusion.

Differential diagnosis of acromegaly

- Pachydermoperiositis syndrome/acromegaloidism
- Phenytoin therapy
- Severe insulin resistance
- Primary hypothyroidism
- Ascher's syndrome
- Multiple neuroma syndrome
- Minoxidil therapy (one case report)

Q. 2 What is the prevalence of acromegaly?

Ans. Acromegaly is an uncommon disorder, with an estimated prevalence of 40–125 per million and an incidence of 3–4 new cases per million.

Q. 3 What are the common presenting clinical features of acromegaly?

Ans. The patients can present with acral enlargement, maxillofacial changes, excessive sweating, arthralgia, headache, hypogonadal symptoms, visual deficit, fatigue, weight gain and galactorrhea in the decreasing order of prevalence (Fig. 1.2).

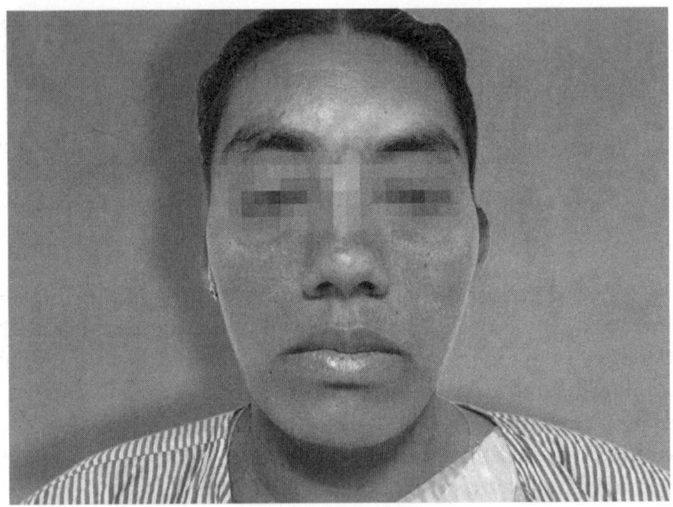

FIG. 1.1 Acromegaly—typical facial features
(For color version, see Plate 1)

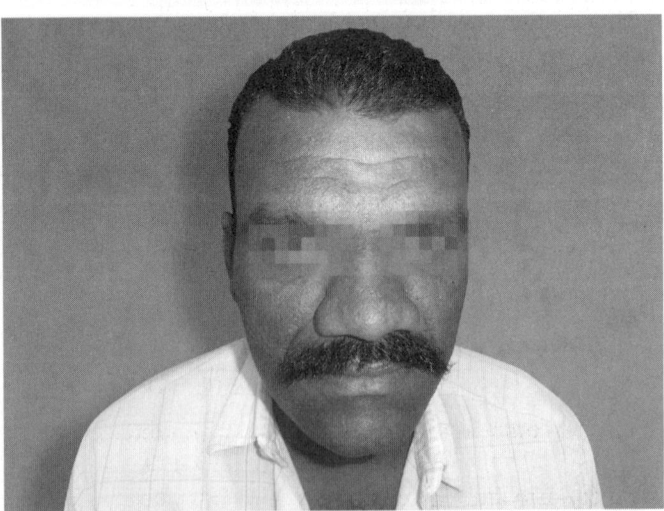

FIG. 1.2 Typical features of acromegaly in a male
(For color version, see Plate 1)

Q. 4 How is a case of acromegaly diagnosed?

Ans. A serum IGF-1 level is good to diagnose, follow-up and monitor a patient with growth hormone excess provided a data of age and sex-matched healthy controls is available.

Q. 5 Is there any use of doing a growth hormone (GH) suppression tests?

Ans. A serum GH level after an oral glucose of 75 g anhydrous can be done, and if the levels measured every 30 minutes for 120 minutes and are less than 1 μg/L, it rules out acromegaly and a level of less than 0.4 ng/mL with ultrasensitive assays.

Q. 6 What is the proposed line of investigation for this patient?

Ans. A growth hormone suppression should be done with 75 g of glucose and IGF-1 levels should also be done. The patient is subjected to a GH suppression test and her post-glucose GH levels are found to be 30 ng/mL and her IGF-1 levels are 800 ng/mL.

Because the most common cause of growth hormone over secretion is a pituitary adenoma. She is subjected to a pituitary MRI which shows a pituitary macroadenoma of 15 mm in size.

Q. 7 Is there an indication for measuring insulin like growth factor binding protein 3 or thyrotropin releasing hormone?

Ans. Presently, there is insufficient data to recommend it routinely and there are no indications to test it.

Q. 8 What imaging investigation should be ordered in this patient?

Ans. Once the diagnosis of acromegaly is confirmed, a pituitary MRI should be performed. A dynamic MRI with contrast will give the best delineation. If the MRI is contraindicated patient may be subjected to CT scan, e.g. if the patient has a pacemaker. It is recommended that the MRI be performed with 2 mm slices to diagnose small microadenomas.

Q. 9 Do we need to do a visual field testing in all patients?

Ans. It should be done, if there is an optic chiasma compression demonstrable on MRI or the patient complains of difficulty in peripheral vision.

Q. 10 Does this patient require any other biochemical testing?

Ans. Further testing is needed to check for hypersecretion of prolactin and also to check for any anterior and posterior pituitary hormones for any evidence of hypopituitarism. The patient is found to have secondary hypothyroidism and ACTH deficiency. Her prolactin levels are normal and her FSH, LH levels are normal. She is started on supplementation with levothyroxine and hydrocortisone.

Q. 11 Does she require any further testing?

Ans. Yes, she needs to be screened for the comorbidities.

Q. 12 What are the comorbidities which have to be targeted?

Ans. Treatment should be directed at the comorbidities, such as aggressive control of lipid abnormalities, type 2 diabetes mellitus, obstructive sleep apnea, arthritic complications, and cardiac dysfunction as well as surveillance for colon polyps.

Q. 13 What are the probable causes of growth hormone excess in this lady?

Ans. Once a biochemical diagnosis of acromegaly has been made, a magnetic resonance imaging (MRI) scan of the pituitary gland (the physician should order a dedicated dynamic pituitary MRI with the use of contrast medium) should be performed because a pituitary GH-secreting adenoma is the cause in most cases.

Q. 14 What is the grading of a pituitary tumor?

Ans. Pituitary tumor can be graded according to the size as microadenoma <10 mm, macroadenoma ≥10 mm and giant adenoma >40 mm by MRI. The tumor can be graded as grade 1a—noninvasive tumor, grade 1b—noninvasive and proliferative tumor, grade 2a—invasive tumor, grade 2b—invasive and proliferative tumor, grade 3—metastatic tumor-cerebrospinal or systemic metastasis.

Q. 15 What should be the ideal assessment of sleep apnea?

Ans. The prevalence of sleep apnea is high (up to 70%) in newly diagnosed patients with acromegaly. Therefore, every patient should have a careful symptomatic assessment (e.g. by Epworth score), and if necessary laboratory assessment, for sleep apnea at the time of diagnosis, in collaboration with a respiratory physician.

Q. 16 How is screening for colonic polyps advised in acromegaly?

Ans. Acromegaly is associated with increased colon polyps and may be associated with increased risk of colorectal cancer, but not cancer mortality (MQ). Colon length may increase during acromegaly resulting in increased mucosal folds known as dolichocolon. It is recommended that a screening colonoscopy be carried out at diagnosis in adults and if negative, then patients should be screened similarly to the general population, especially if insulin-like growth factor-I (IGF-I) levels are normalized. If IGF-I remains persistently elevated, more frequent screening is recommended (SR). If colonoscopy is abnormal, follow-up and screening should be in accordance with clinical guidelines.

Q. 17 What complications need to be screened in acromegaly?

Ans. The following routine baseline assessments are therefore required for patients with acromegaly: electrocardiogram (ECG), echocardiogram, blood pressure measurement, and the Epworth scale or sleep study for sleep apnea. These patients also require assessment of the peripheral arterial system.

Q. 18 What is new in the genetics of acromegaly?

Ans. A recurrent activating *GPR101* mutation (p.E308D) has been shown in 11 of 248 tumor DNA samples from patients with isolated acromegaly. Of these patients, 3 carried a germline *GPR101* mutation. This might suggest a higher prevalence of germline *GPR101* mutation among patients with sporadic acromegaly.

Q. 19 What is familial acromegaly?

Ans. Familial acromegaly is generally diagnosed at an earlier age than nonfamilial acromegaly and young patients (<30 years old) with aggressive acromegaly, or individuals with a family member who has a pituitary tumor, should be considered for genetic screening for markers of familial acromegaly (DR). Carney complex, familial isolated pituitary adenoma (FIPA) and multiple endocrine neoplasia type 1 should be considered. An increased awareness that FIPA is associated with mutations in the aryl hydrocarbon receptor interacting protein (AIP) gene is required.

Q. 20 What are the options for treatment available for this patient?

Ans. This patient should be offered surgery because that can provide complete and early cure and normalization of the growth hormone levels.

If the tumor is large then the options of surgical versus initial medical therapy can be discussed with the patient and also cost factor should be discussed if the patient is planning for medical therapy.

Appropriate patients can be told about option of radiotherapy.

The patient undergoes a transsphenoidal resection of the pituitary tumor and she is given a stress dose of hydrocortisone in view of the preoperative diagnosis of cortisol deficiency.

Q. 21 What are the recommendations for checking the growth hormone levels after surgery for acromegaly?

Ans. Following surgery, it is suggested measuring an IGF-1 level and a random GH at 12 weeks or later. It also suggests measuring a nadir GH level after a glucose load in a patient with a GH greater than 1 µg/L.

Although GH testing may be performed as early as postoperative day 1, the role of an immediate postoperative GH value may be limited, because an elevated value may reflect surgical stress with normal somatotroph GH production. The decline in IGF-1 is more delayed compared with GH, likely due to differential half-life of IGF-binding proteins.

If the IGF-1 level has declined but is still not normal, measurement of a repeat IGF-1 level is warranted due to variability in the IGF-1 assay.

Serum IGF-1 levels should be repeated at 12 weeks after surgery and a normal level suggests surgical cure but if the levels do not show a normal value post 12 weeks then a repeat level should be checked again at 9–11 weeks to check for a delayed normalization of values. The fallacy of IGF-1 level ranges not being the same in different population subsets and lack of normative data for our population has to be kept in mind when interpreting the results of IGF-1.

Q. 22 What value of growth hormone after oral glucose tolerance test (OGTT) is considered as normal?

Ans. A value of growth hormone of less than 1 ng/mL, suggests a complete cure but a value of 0.4 ng/mL may increase the sensitivity of testing.

Q. 23 When should a repeat MRI be done for pituitary postoperative?

Ans. It should be done at 12 weeks after surgery to see for the size of residual tumor.

This patient in case 1 undergoes a postoperative evaluation for pituitary hormones after 6 weeks of surgery and she is found to have secondary hypothyroidism and cortisol deficiency. Her postoperative GH levels are 8 ng/mL (growth hormone suppression test) and her IGF-1 levels are 360 ng/mL at 12 weeks post surgery. Her pituitary MRI shows a small residual lesion of 6 mm in size which is done after 12 weeks of surgery.

Q. 24 What are the recommendations for postoperative monitoring of these hormones?

Ans. Postoperatively patients need to be monitored for diabetes insipidus and SIADH for 2 weeks.

Q. 25 What options of medical therapy are available?

Ans. The options of medical therapy are dopamine agonists, SSAs, and a GH receptor antagonist.

Q. 26 What options of dopamine agonists are available?

Ans. They may be considered as first line in patients who have financial constraints. The commonly used dopamine agonist is cabergoline. Dopamine agonists may be considered particularly in patients with mild biochemical activity, such as in the setting of modestly elevated serum IGF-I levels in the absence or concomitant presence of somatostatin analog (SSA) therapy.

Q. 27 Are dopamine agonists more efficacious in patients with hyperprolactinemia?

Ans. The studies have not shown that the response is better in patients with concomitant hyperprolactinemia.

Q. 28 What options of somatostatin analogs are available?

Ans. Somatostatin analogs (SSAs) are effective in normalizing IGF-I and GH levels in approximately 55% of patients. The clinical and biochemical responses to SSAs are inversely related to tumor size and degree of GH hypersecretion. Octreotide long-acting release (LAR) and lanreotide autogel have similar efficacy profiles.

Q. 29 What is the status of pasireotide in the treatment of acromegaly?

Ans. Pasireotide is a new pan somatostatin receptor ligand with binding affinity to somatostatin receptors subtype 5 SST5 > SST2 > SST3 > SST1. It has been shown to cause suppression of GH levels to less than 2.5 ng/mL and normalization of insulin like growth factor 1 in one-thirds of patients with acromegaly.

Q. 30 Do somatostatin analogs have any effect on the tumor size?

Ans. They reduce pituitary tumor size modestly in approximately 25–70% of patients, depending on whether they are used as adjuvant or *de novo* therapy.

Q. 31 Should all patients with acromegaly receive somatostatin analog therapy before surgery?

Ans. No current guidelines do not recommend the routine use of somatostatin analog pretreatment prior to surgery in patients with growth hormone-secreting pituitary tumors.

Q. 32 Is regular radiologic investigation in patients with dopamine agonists to screen for gallbladder disease required for these patients?

Ans. No, it is not warranted. Only clinical symptoms need to be asked for.

Q. 33 What is the status of GH receptor antagonist treatment?

Ans. Pegvisomant is a GH receptor antagonist that competes with endogenous GH for its receptor and prevents functional dimerization and signal transduction by the GH receptor.

It is highly effective in reducing growth hormone levels in patients who are resistant to other forms of therapy. Pegvisomant is highly effective in normalizing IGF-I values (>90%), including patients who are partially or completely resistant to other medical therapies.

> Do not monitor a patient on pegvisomant with growth hormone levels.

Q. 34 What is the disease recommendation for pegvisomant?

Ans. It is administered as a daily subcutaneous injection though other regimes are recommended including twice a week or once a week.

Q. 35 What monitoring is needed when patient is on pegvisomant?

Ans. Patients should be counseled about the side effects of pegvisomant, including flu-like illness, allergic reactions, and increase in liver enzymes. Therefore, serial monitoring of results of liver function tests (LFTs) is suggested at monthly intervals for the first 6 months, quarterly for the next 6 months, and then biannually. Patients with elevated baseline results of LFTs need more frequent monitoring.

Q. 36 What is the status of combination therapy?

Ans. In patients with inadequate response to somatostatin analogs combination therapy may be advocated with cabergoline for better biochemical response.

Q. 37 What are the options of radiotherapy?

Ans. Pituitary radiotherapy may be offered to patients who have not achieved complete cure with surgical and medical therapy.

Q. 38 What type of radiotherapy is preferred?

Ans. Because of the technical advances and convenience stereotactic radiosurgery may be considered the preferred mode of RT over conventional RT in patients with acromegaly, unless the technique is not available, there is substantial residual tumor burden, or the tumor is too close (<5 mm) to the optic chiasma.

Q. 39 What are the goals of treatment in acromegaly?

Ans. It includes normalization of growth hormone and IGF-1 levels.

She is given the option of radiotherapy and medical therapy. The patient does not want to go for radiotherapy or for repeat surgery and she opts for medical therapy. She is started on octreotide LAR once in 28 days intramuscular injection and is asked to follow-up.

Q. 40 What is surgical remission?

Ans. A serum GH <0.14 mg/L suggests surgical remission, and a level <1 mg/L indicates control and normalization of the mortality risk.

Drug	*Dose*
SRL	
Octreotide	50–400 g SC every 8 hour
Octreotide LAR	10–40 mg IM every 4 weeks
Lanreotide	30 mg IM every 10–14 days
Lanreotide autogel	60–129 mg deep SC every 4 weeks
GH antagonist	
Pegvisomant	10–40 mg SC daily
Dopamine agonist	
Cabergoline	1–4 mg orally every week

CASE 2

A woman 31 years of age who is a follow-up case of acromegaly comes to the endocrinology outpatient department for follow-up. She was operated about 5 years back after which she was subjected to radiotherapy because of the residual lesion and persistently high postoperative growth hormone levels of 10 ng/mL and high levels of IGF-1. She is now four years post-radiotherapy and has come for follow-up. She has IGF-1 levels of and post-glucose growth hormone levels of 5 ng/mL. She has regular menstrual cycles and has got married. She wants to now plan for pregnancy and wants an opinion, if she can go ahead. She has a cycle with intermenstrual distance of 30 days and her 23rd day's progesterone levels are 0.1 ng/mL. What should she be advised now?

Q. 1 What is the management of hypogonadism in postoperative cases of acromegaly?

Ans. The hypogonadism is seen in 50% of the patients and is reversible. The biochemical diagnosis in males may be difficult, due to low sex hormone-binding globulin levels, thus making interpretation of total testosterone values more challenging. In these circumstances, assessment of clinical symptoms and bioavailable testosterone are important for diagnosis. Concomitant hyperprolactinemia should be considered as a cause of hypogonadism. Treatment of hypogonadism is done as it is done in a nonacromegaly patient. The females can be diagnosed easily.

Factors predicting suboptimal response and disease persistence after treatment for acromegaly

- Younger age at diagnosis
- High expression of tumor aggression markers such as Ki67, p53 and pituitary tumor transforming gene (PTTG)
- Sparsely granulated adenomas
- Hyperintense imaging on T2-weighted magnetic resonance imaging
- Very large adenomas and actively growing tumors
- No previous radiation therapy, especially during pegvisomant therapy
- Previous, suboptimal response to SRL therapy
- High GH and IGF-I levels during long-term follow-up
- Larger tumor remnants after surgery

Q. 2 What should be done in pregnancy?

Ans. The biochemical monitoring with GH levels and IGF-1 levels is of limited use in pregnancy.

Q. 3 Should we regularly do MRI in pregnancy?

Ans. MRI scan should not be routinely performed in pregnancy unless there is a new or worsening visual compromise.

The woman in the present case is subjected to ovulation induction. She conceives, and there is no visual compromise documented during the pregnancy. Postoperatively, she breastfeeds the child but her postdelivery growth hormone levels are high so after breastfeeding is stopped, she is given the option of radiotherapy and somatostatin analog therapy. She opts for somatostatin analog therapy and she is continuing on it and her present GH levels are 2 ng/mL as compared to the pretreatment levels of 8 ng/mL after 6 months of somatostatin analog therapy.

CASE 3

A boy 18 years of age is brought with progressively increasing height and increase in shoe size. The child also complains of headache and banging onto objects on side frequently for past 4 months. The same has been noticed by the parents. The parents feel that the child should have stopped growing fast by now as his siblings are much shorter than him though they are older.

On examination, the child's height was 187 cm and his two older brothers were 168 and 169 cm each and his midparental height was 165 cm. The child was subjected to a growth hormone suppression test with 75 g glucose and his growth hormone levels at 60 and 120 minutes were respectively 20 ng/mL and 22 ng/mL. His IGF-1 levels were much higher as compared to his age.

He was then subjected to a dynamic MRI of pituitary with contrast and it showed a macroadenoma of the pituitary impinging on the optic chiasma.

The child was subjected to a visual field testing which showed bilateral hemianopia.

Associated syndromes with gigantism	Differential diagnosis of gigantism
• Multiple endocrine neoplasia (MEN) type I • McCune-Albright syndrome • Neurofibromatosis • Tuberous sclerosis • Carney complex	• Familial tall stature • Beckwith-Wiedemann syndrome • Cerebral gigantism (Sotos syndrome): From *NSD1* gene mutation or other causes • Weaver syndrome • Estrogen receptor mutation • Simpson-Golabi-Behmel syndrome

The child is planned for surgery.

The postoperative growth hormone levels are found to be 4 ng/mL and IGF-1 continues to be high. Hence, the option of medical therapy is discussed with the parents. In view of the financial constraints the child is planned for dopamine agonist therapy in form of cabergoline 0.5 mg twice a week.

The child is subsequently followed up.

Q. 1 What is gigantism?

Ans. Gigantism is a non-specific term that denotes excessive growth in a pediatric patient. This may over production of growth hormone (GH) being the cause of gigantism is rare and is termed *pituitary gigantism*, or it may arise from an overgrowth syndrome. Pituitary gigantism can present as early as during infancy or not until adolescence, and may be congenital or acquired. It may occur as a sporadic condition or in the context of a well-described syndrome in which hypersecretion of GH is a potential feature.

Q. 2 What are the causes of growth hormone excess in children?

Ans. Conditions in which GH excess occurs include Neurofibromatosis type 1, McCune-Albright syndrome, Multiple endocrine neoplasia type 1, Carney complex, Isolated familial somatotropinomas and X-linked acrogigantism.

Q. 3 What are the different overgrowth syndromes in children which are not due to growth hormone secreting tumors?

Ans. These include Sotos syndrome, Beckwith-Wiedemann syndrome, Simpson-Golabi-Behmel syndrome and Weaver syndrome.

Q. 4 What approach is different in children with gigantism?

Ans. The modality of radiotherapy is not preferred in children with gigantism but other treatment modalities and follow-up remain the same. The patients with gigantism particularly need to be screened for vascular disease including peripheral vascular disease.

Q. 5 What is the most cost-effective approach versus more value added approach for the treatment of acromegaly?

Ans. The value of surgery as first-line therapy for patients with surgically accessible lesions is not debatable. Surgery provides the greatest value for management of patients with acromegaly. However, in accordance with the

Acromegaly Consensus Group's recent recommendations, somatostatin analogs provide the greatest value and should be used as first-line therapy for patients who cannot be managed surgically.

SUGGESTED READING

1. Bolanowski M, Halupczok J, Jawiarczyk-Przybyłowska A. Pituitary disorders and osteoporosis. Int J Endocrinol. 2015;2015:206853. doi: 10.1155/2015/206853. Epub 2015 Mar 19. Review.
2. Carroll PV, Jenkins PJ. Acromegaly. In: De Groot LJ, Beck-Peccoz P, Chrousos G, Dungan K, Grossman A, Hershman JM, Koch C, McLachlan R, New M, Rebar R, Singer F, Vinik A, Weickert MO (Eds), 2012 Endotext [Internet]. South Dartmouth (MA): MDText.com, Inc. 2000.
3. Dutta P, Hajela A, Pathak A, Bhansali A, Radotra BD, Vashishta RK, et al. Clinical profile and outcome of patients with acromegaly according to the 2014 consensus guidelines: Impact of a multi-disciplinary team. NeurolIndia. 2015;63(3):360-8.
4. Eugster E. Gigantism. In: De Groot LJ, Beck-Peccoz P, Chrousos G, Dungan K, Grossman A, Hershman JM, Koch C, McLachlan R, New M, Rebar R, Singer F, Vinik A, Weickert MO (Eds), 2015 Endotext [Internet]. South Dartmouth (MA):MDText.com, Inc. 2000.
5. Giustina A, Chanson P, Kleinberg D, Bronstein MD, Clemmons DR, Klibanski A, et al. Acromegaly Consensus Group. Expert consensus document: a consensus on the medical treatment of acromegaly. Nat Rev Endocrinol. 2014;10(4):243-8.
6. Jacob JJ, Bevan JS. Should all patients with acromegaly receive somatostatin analogue therapy before surgery and, if so, for how long? Clin Endocrinol (Oxf). 2014;81(6): 812-7.
7. Kamenický P, Bouligand J, Chanson P. Gigantism, acromegaly, and GPR101 mutations. N Engl J Med. 2015;372(13):1264.
8. Katznelson L, Laws ER Jr, Melmed S, Molitch ME, Murad MH, Utz A, et al. Endocrine Society. Acromegaly: an endocrine society clinical practice guideline. J Clin Endocrinol Metab. 2014;99(11):3933-51. doi: 10.1210/jc.2014-2700. Epub. 2014 Oct 30.
9. Kimmell KT, Weil RJ, Marko NF. Multi-modal management of acromegaly: a value perspective. Pituitary. 2015 Jan 4. [Epub ahead of print] PubMed PMID: 25557288.
10. Lois K, Bukowczan J, Perros P, Jones S, Gunn M, James RA. The role of colonoscopic screening in acromegaly revisited: review of current literature and practice guidelines. Pituitary. 2014 Jul 23. [Epub ahead of print] Störmann S, Schopohl J. Emerging drugs for acromegaly. Expert Opin Emerg Drugs. 2014;19(1):79-97.
11. Melmed S, Casanueva FF, Klibanski A, Bronstein MD, Chanson P, Lamberts SW, et al. A consensus on the diagnosis and treatment of acromegaly complications. Pituitary. 2013;16(3):294-302.
12. Störmann S, Schopohl J. Emerging drugs for acromegaly. Expert Opin Emerg Drugs. 2014;19(1):79-97. doi: 10.1517/14728214.2014.875529. Epub 2013 Dec 28.Review.
13. Syro LV, Rotondo F, Kovacs K. Biomarkers of acromegaly. Endocrine. 2015;49(1):4-5. doi: 10.1007/s12020-015-0579-9. Epub 2015 Mar 18.
14. Verrua E, Ferrante E, Filopanti M, Malchiodi E, Sala E, Giavoli C, et al. Reevaluation of acromegalic patients in long-term remission according to newly proposed consensus criteria for control of disease. Int J Endocrinol. 2014;2014:581-94. doi: 10.1155/2014/581594. Epub 2014 Dec 21.

CHAPTER

2

Cushing's Disease: Contemporary Diagnosis and Management

Madhukar Mittal, Satyendra Sonkar, Pradyut Tiwari

CASE

A 29-year-old female presented with progressive swelling over the body, weight gain, menstrual irregularity. On examination, her BP was 160/100 mm Hg, pulse rate 86/min, weight 88 kg, height 155 cm. Buffalo hump was present with broad purplish striae over the abdomen. Proximal muscle weakness was present. Her investigations revealed Hb 12.6 g%, fasting blood sugar (FBS) 170 mg%, creatinine 0.9, Na 140 mEq/L, K 3.4 mEq/L (Fig. 2.1).

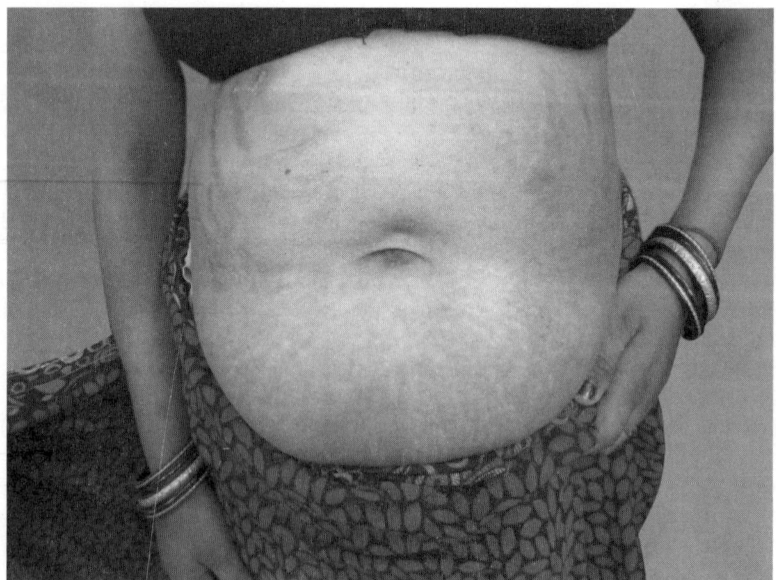

FIG. 2.1 Striae of Cushing's syndrome
(For color version, see Plate 2)

Q. 1 How would you approach a case of suspected Cushing's syndrome?

Ans. Step 1—rule out exogenous Cushing's by history of drug (steroid) intake
Step 2—rule out pseudo-Cushing's by clinical evaluation and screening tests
Step 3—perform diagnostic tests for confirming endogenous Cushing's syndrome
Step 4—perform tests for finding out possible cause of Cushing's
Step 5—radiological investigations for localizing tumor (Flowchart 2.1).

Table 2.1 listed the various tests for screening.

Two screening tests are recommended for confirming hypercortisolism taking into consideration their sensitivity and specificity, and also the availability.

> Dexamethasone is used for suppression testing because, unlike prednisolone, it does not cross-react in radioimmunoassay for cortisol.

The interpretation of the results depends upon the assay used and the local laboratory calibration.

- These assays differ widely in their accuracy and the values near the cut-off value close to the functional limit of detection should be interpreted carefully as precision deteriorates at the lower levels.
- There are many drugs and conditions which can interfere with the measurement of cortisol and while interpreting, the physician should be aware of these limitations. Drugs like estrogen containing pills, increase cortisol binding globulin and thereby cause false positive results.
- Sensitivity and specificity of the various tests depend upon the cut-off value that was taken.
- In the case of any equivocal results, rescreening may be required.

FLOWCHART 2.1 Suspected Cushing's syndrome: Clinical features

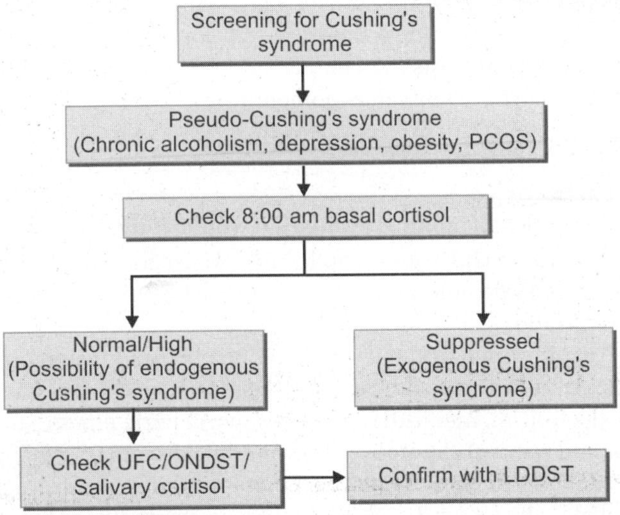

Screening for Cushing's syndrome
↓
Pseudo-Cushing's syndrome (Chronic alcoholism, depression, obesity, PCOS)
↓
Check 8:00 am basal cortisol
↓
- Normal/High (Possibility of endogenous Cushing's syndrome)
  ↓
  Check UFC/ONDST/ Salivary cortisol → Confirm with LDDST
- Suppressed (Exogenous Cushing's syndrome)

Abbreviations: LDDST, low-dose dexamethasone suppression test; ONDST, overnight dexamethasone suppression test; PCOS, polycystic ovary syndrome; UFC, urinary free cortisol

TABLE 2.1 Screening/Diagnostic tests

Test	*Method*	*Value*	*Sensitivity*	*Specificity*	*Comments*
ONDST	1 mg dexamethasone the night before collection	>1.8 μg/dL	98–100%	88%	For screening. Easy to perform on OPD basis
UFC	24-hour urine collection	>100 μg/24 hours	95–100%	90–95%	More than 2–4 times upper limit suggests Cushing's syndrome
Salivary cortisol	Midnight saliva	>0.27 μg/dL (midnight)	100%	96%	Convenient and noninvasive
Midnight cortisol	Midnight serum	>7.5 μg/dL (awake)	94%	100%	Take care to avoid stress
LDDST	0.5 mg dexamethasone every 6 hrs for 48 hours	>1.8 μg/dL	98–100%	97–100%	Diagnostic of endogenous Cushing's syndrome

Abbreviations: LDDST, low-dose dexamethasone suppression test; ONDST, overnight dexamethasone suppression test; UFC, urinary free cortisol

As exogenous Cushing's syndrome is more common than the endogenous one, exclusion of this condition is very important. In iatrogenic Cushing's syndrome, cortisol levels are low unless the patient is taking a corticosteroid (such as prednisolone), which may cross-react in radioimmunoassay of cortisol. Apart from the history, basal 8:00 AM cortisol value will differentiate the exogenous from the endogenous Cushing's syndrome. A suppressed cortisol value with Cushingoid features suggests exogenous cause except for cyclical Cushing's syndrome which can have low values sometimes.

Q. 2 What are the causes of Cushing's syndrome?

Ans. See Box 2.1.

Q. 3. What other relevant clinical evaluation would you like to do?

Ans. We would like to check for complications of excessive steroid and rule out pseudo-Cushing's syndrome and take treatment history regarding exogenous steroid administration.

Pseudo-Cushing's syndrome is characterized by mild hypercortisolism and may be difficult to distinguish from true Cushing's syndrome. Causes include depression, alcoholism, medications, obesity, psychiatric illness, stress/trauma/acute illness, and states of elevated cortisol-binding protein (pregnancy, estrogen therapy). Pseudo-Cushing's syndrome may produce results suggestive of hypercortisolism, abnormal dexamethasone suppressibility and mild elevation of urinary free cortisol (UFC). The distinguishing feature of this disorder is that

BOX 2.1 Etiology of Cushing's syndrome

Adrenocorticotropic hormone (ACTH)-dependent causes:
- Cushing's disease (pituitary adenoma) 70%
- Ectopic
  - ACTH syndrome 5–10% (bronchial carcinoid, small-cell lung CA and other neuroendocrine tumor)
  - Corticotropin-releasing hormone (CRH) syndrome (rare)
- Ectopic corticotropin-releasing hormone (CRH) syndrome (rare)
- Macronodular adrenal hyperplasia <5%

ACTH-independent causes:
- Iatrogenic—Most common cause
- Adrenal adenoma (10%)
- Adrenal carcinoma (5–10%)
- PPNAD <5%
- Carney's syndrome <5%
- McCune-Albright syndrome (rare)
- Aberrant receptor expression [GIP, IL-1b (rare)]

Pseudo-Cushing's syndromes:
- Excessive alcohol intake
- Major depressive disorder
- Obesity
- PCOS

Abbreviations: GIP, gastric inhibitory polypeptide; PPNAD, primary pigmented nodular adrenal hyperplasia; PCOS, polycystic ovary syndrome

the laboratory and clinical findings of hypercortisolism disappear if the primary process is successfully treated. The metabolic syndrome which is characterized by central obesity, hypertension, and glucose intolerance may mimic Cushing's syndrome. The polycystic ovarian syndrome may present with menstrual irregularities and hyperandrogenism (hirsutism, acne) similar to features of Cushing's syndrome.

Q. 4 What investigations would you like to do to confirm your diagnosis?

Ans. Two days low dose dexamethasone suppression test is used for diagnosis. Other tests which are supportively used for diagnosis include 24-hour urine free cortisol, midnight cortisol, salivary cortisol (Box 2.1).

Q. 5 How do you further investigate a patient of Cushing's syndrome?

Ans. The next line involves two critical steps:

1. Determining, if the cortisol excess is ACTH independent or ACTH dependent (Does the patient have primary adrenal disease or an ACTH-secreting tumor?)
2. If ACTH secreting, then determining the source of the ACTH in the ACTH-dependent form (Does the patient have Cushing's disease (pituitary adenoma) or ectopic ACTH syndrome?)

Measurement of ACTH

Adrenocorticotropic hormone (ACTH) measurement will help us to differentiate ACTH from the non-ACTH-dependent Cushing's syndrome. Sample is collected with adequate precautions in the morning at 9:00 AM and measured. Some centers advocate checking the ACTH in the midnight along with the cortisol to interpret and differentiate the two. Morning ACTH value of less than 10 pg/mL is suggestive of an ACTH-independent Cushing's syndrome. And the value of more than 22 pg/mL is suggestive of ACTH-dependent Cushing's syndrome. Further testing is required, if the values are equivocal. Patients with equivocal ACTH values between 10 and 20 pg/mL may be subjected to corticotropin-releasing hormone (CRH) stimulation test and the increment of the ACTH and cortisol response are suggestive of Cushing's disease.

High-dose dexamethasone suppression test (HDDST) though used to differentiate the pituitary from ectopic ACTH-dependent Cushing's syndrome is not definitive. The sensitivity and the specificity depend on the amount of cortisol suppression, and can be suppressed in carcinoid syndrome producing ACTH.

Other tests that are available to differentiate the cause of Cushing's syndrome are given in Table 2.2.

- Adrenocorticotropic hormone values between 10 and 20 pg/mL are subjected to the CRH stimulation to differentiate, but the clinical clues such as pigmentation and imaging have to be considered before coming to a conclusion. Although many tests are available, none of them clearly differentiate the patients with equivocal results. Therefore, a lot of clinical discretion is required and the treating endocrinologist should also be aware of all the pitfalls of the diagnostic tests.
- Adrenocorticotropic hormone molecule is rapidly degraded by the plasma proteases. Hence, it should be collected in a prechilled tube to avoid false low values. So while interpreting the value, ensure proper collection of the sample.

TABLE 2.2 Used to differentiate origin of Cushing's syndrome

Test	*Method*	*Value*	*Sensitivity*	*Specificity*	*Comments*
CRH test	1 µg of ovine or human CRH	ACTH >35% Cortisol >20%	93% (for ACTH)	100% (for cortisol)	Used to diagnose Cushing's disease
HDDST	2 mg for 48 hours	>90% suppression of basal 8:00 am cortisol	67–70%	100%	Not completely definitive
BIPSS	Bilateral inferior petrosal sinus sampling	Basal central: Peripheral 2:1 CRH stimulated >3:1	95%	100%	Used to differentiate pituitary versus ectopic

Abbreviations: CRH, corticotropin releasing hormone; HDDST, high-dose dexamethasone suppression test; BIPSS, bilateral inferior petrosal sinus sampling

- High-dose dexamethasone suppression test shows suppression by only less than 50% of the basal cortisol value in about 80% of the patients with Cushing's disease. And there are high numbers of false positive tests (10–30%) in ectopic Cushing's syndrome.

Q. 6 What could be other problems/complications associated with Cushing's disease?

Ans. *Progressive central obesity* involving the abdomen, face, and neck (buffalo hump, moon facies, supraclavicular fat pads, and exophthalmos from retro-orbital fat deposition).

Metabolic complications include glucose intolerance (owing to stimulation of gluconeogenesis by cortisol and peripheral insulin resistance caused by obesity), and hypertension (through poorly understood multifactorial etiologies), both of which confer increased cardiovascular risk, a major cause of morbidity and death in patients with Cushing's syndrome. Severe hypertension and hypokalemia are more commonly seen in patients with ectopic ACTH syndrome because the very high serum cortisol levels overwhelm the capacity of the 11-β-hydroxysteroid dehydrogenase type 2 enzyme, which oxidizes cortisol to inactive cortisone in renal tubules, thereby resulting in activation of mineralocorticoid receptors, hence causing hypokalemic alkalosis. Hypokalemia aggravates hyperglycemia by inhibiting insulin secretion.

Dermatologic manifestations include skin atrophy (thinning of the stratum corneum), hair thinning, fragile skin with easy bruisability, wide purple striae (due to the stretching of fragile skin), cutaneous fungal infections, and hyperpigmentation (in ectopic ACTH syndrome).

Reproductive changes include menstrual irregularities, hirsutism, oily facial skin with acne, and other signs of virilization (temporal balding, deepening voice), especially in women with adrenal carcinoma.

Musculoskeletal manifestations are proximal myopathy, muscle wasting (resulting from the catabolic effects of excess glucocorticoid on skeletal muscle as well as aggravated due to resulting hypokalemia), and osteoporosis (caused by decreased bone formation, increased bone resorption, and decreased intestinal and renal calcium reabsorption). Vertebral compression fractures, pathologic fractures of the rib or long bones, and aseptic necrosis of the femoral heads may also be present.

Neuropsychiatric changes can include labile mood, agitated depression, anxiety, panic attacks, mild paranoia, impaired short-term memory and cognition, and insomnia.

- Clinical features which are more common in exogenous Cushing's syndrome are glaucoma, cataract, benign intracranial hypertension, pancreatitis and avascular necrosis of the head of the femur.
- Cushing's syndrome is more likely, if onset of above feature is at a young age.

It is to be noted spontaneous Cushing's syndrome is rare, and hence the positive predictive value of any one feature alone is low.

In malignant ACTH secreting tumor, there may be cachexia with rapid presentation in comparison to a benign tumor.

In Cushing's disease, there is usually micropituitary adenoma <10 mm in diameter, and hence visual loss is not present.

Q. 7 What imaging would be required in Cushing's syndrome?

Ans. Once the diagnosis of ACTH or non-ACTH-dependent Cushing's syndrome is made appropriate imaging is done. In non-ACTH-dependent Cushing's CT/MRI of the adrenal gland is done but CT gives the better resolution of the adrenal anatomy.

In ACTH-dependent Cushing's syndrome, the first step is to image the pituitary, and see if there is any abnormality and for this MRI of the pituitary is done with gadolinium enhancement. Use of dynamic MRI (with IV gadolinium) sequences increases the sensitivity of detection. However, caution has to be exercised in diagnosing microadenomas as the possibility of an incidentaloma is as high as 10% in general population.

If the pituitary imaging is negative, then imaging of the thorax, abdomen head and neck has to be done to detect the ectopic source of production of the ACTH [mostly thymoma, carcinoid, pheochromocytoma, medullary thyroid carcinoma (MTC) or malignancy]. In patients with suspected ectopic ACTH and not localized, special imaging like 18F-fluorodeoxyglucose positron emission tomography (FDG-PET) may be done.

Inferior petrosal sinus sampling (IPSS) is an invasive procedure that involves measuring the central-to-peripheral ACTH gradient and may be useful when the source of ACTH production (i.e. pituitary versus ectopic) remains elusive despite other noninvasive testing [i.e. when there is cortisol suppression on HDDST (suggesting Cushing's disease) in the setting of a negative pituitary MRI].

Q. 8 What are the treatment modalities for Cushing's syndrome?

Ans.

- Treatment is based on the source of the hypercortisolism, so the need for an accurate diagnosis cannot be overemphasized. The goal of treatment is to reverse the clinical manifestations of hypercortisolemia by decreasing cortisol secretion to normal levels.
- *In exogenous Cushing's syndrome,* gradual withdrawal of the glucocorticoid is important because most patients on long-term therapy will have some degree of HPA-axis suppression with resultant adrenal insufficiency if therapy is abruptly discontinued.
- *In ACTH-independent Cushing's syndrome,* adrenal imaging by either CT or MRI will demonstrate unilateral or bilateral disease. Patients should be referred for *adrenalectomy*. During and after unilateral adrenalectomy, patients should receive glucocorticoid replacement until the HPA axis recovers from the prolonged suppressive effects of glucocorticoid excess. Patients with bilateral adrenalectomy require lifelong glucocorticoid and mineralocorticoid replacement.
- *In Cushing's disease, a trans-sphenoidal pituitary surgery* is the treatment of choice for patients with a clearly circumscribed microadenoma. In other cases, subtotal resection of the anterior pituitary may be performed. Patients with

incomplete resection of the tumor may undergo repeat surgery or pituitary irradiation with either conventional radiation or stereotactic radiation with the gamma knife. Pituitary irradiation may not control the hypercortisolemia for months to years, and patients require medical therapy until the full effects of the radiation take effect. Surgical cure with transsphenoidal adenomectomy can be assessed on postoperative day 2–3 with morning cortisol levels, which are undetectable with successful complete resection of the tumor. After transsphenoidal resection of the adenoma, patients require glucocorticoid replacement until recovery of the HPA axis (Table 2.3).
- *Ectopic ACTH-dependent Cushing's syndrome* should be confirmed with imaging studies, including CT, MRI, and/or scintigraphy. Tumors that can be localized by imaging studies should be removed surgically. If the source is an occult tumor or if there is metastatic disease, medical treatment is required. Bilateral adrenalectomy may be performed in refractory cases.

Surgery

- Preferred treatment modality
- Trans-sphenoidal pituitary resection.

Medical Management

Following are the indications for medical management in Cushing's syndrome:
- Preoperatively to control cortisol levels
- Patients in whom surgery is contraindicated
- Patients in whom surgery/radiotherapy has failed
- Awaiting effect of radiotherapy to take place
- *Ketoconazole* is an antifungal agent that inhibits 17, 20-lyase, 11-β-hydroxylase, and cholesterol side-chain cleavage enzyme. It is usually the first-line medication. Its cortisol-reducing effects are dose-dependent and can be seen rapidly. The major side effect is liver toxicity. Other side effects include gynecomastia, impotence, and gastrointestinal symptoms. Doses range from 200 to 1200 mg orally daily in 2–3 divided doses.

TABLE 2.3 Medical therapy of Cushing's syndrome

Inhibit steroidogenesis	Metyrapone Ketoconazole	Days to weeks	Cause GI side effects and ketoconazole cause insufficiency
Inhibits glucocorticoid receptor	Mifepristone Etomidate	Days	Etomidate can be used for acute control
Modulate ACTH release	Cabergoline Octreotide Pasireotide	Months	Effect may be variable and slow
Adrenolytic	Mitotane	Days to weeks	Can cause adrenal insufficiency

- *Mitotane* inhibits cholesterol side-chain cleavage enzyme and 11-β-hydroxylase. Mitotane induces permanent destruction of adrenocortical cells and, therefore, can be used to achieve medical adrenalectomy as an alternative to surgical adrenalectomy. Glucocorticoid replacement is started at initiation of mitotane treatment. Mineralocorticoid treatment may eventually be required. Side effects are generally dose dependent and include gastrointestinal symptoms, weakness, lethargy, leukopenia, gynecomastia, and hypercholesterolemia. Doses start at 0.5 g orally at bedtime and are increased slowly to 2–3 g/day in 3 to 4 divided doses for a total of 6–9 months.
- *Metyrapone* inhibits 11-β-hydroxylase. Major side effects include increased androgens, hypertension, and hypokalemia through increased 11-deoxycorticosterone. Doses range from 250 to 1000 mg orally, given every 6 hours. Lower doses of 500–750 mg orally daily can be used when given in combination with ketoconazole and/or aminoglutethimide.
- *Aminoglutethimide* is an anticonvulsant that inhibits the cholesterol side-chain cleavage enzyme. The usual dose is 250 mg 2–3 times a day. Side effects include gastrointestinal upset, lethargy, ataxia, hypothyroidism, headache, bone marrow suppression, and skin rash. It is not as effective for monotherapy as ketoconazole or metyrapone, and thus is frequently used in combination with other agents.
- Other agents with limited or modest anticorticosteroid capabilities include Mifepristone (RU486), somatostatin receptor ligands (octreotide, lanreotide, pasireotide), Etomidate, and dopamine receptor agonists (bromocriptine or cabergoline).

Radiotherapy

Indication: Residual disease after initial pituitary surgery.

Fractionated external beam radiotherapy or stereotactic radiosurgery achieves control of hypercortisolism in approximately 50–60% of patients within 3–5 year. Long-term follow-up is necessary to detect relapse, which can occur after an initial response to both types of radiotherapy. The incidence of therapy-induced pituitary failure appears to be similar with radiotherapy or radiosurgery. Insufficient studies are available to evaluate the effects of radiotherapy on cerebrovascular and neurocognitive functions. The risk of second tumor formation after pituitary radiation is considered to be in the range of 1–2%.

SUGGESTED READING

1. Barnett R. Cushing's syndrome. Lancet. 2016;388(10045):649.
2. Bronstein MD, Machado MC, Fragoso MC. Management of endocrine disease: Management of pregnant patients with Cushing's syndrome. Eur J Endocrinol. 2015;173(2):R85-91. doi: 10.1530/EJE-14-1130. Review. PubMed PMID: 25872515.
3. Li LL, Dou JT, Yang GQ, Gu WJ, Lü ZH, Mu YM. Etiology analysis of 522 hospitalized cases with Cushing syndrome. Zhonghua Yi Xue Za Zhi. 2016;96(31):2454-7.

4. Nieman LK. Cushing's syndrome: update on signs, symptoms and biochemical screening. Eur J Endocrinol. 2015;173(4):M33-8. doi: 10.1530/EJE-15-0464.Review.
5. Santhanam P, Taieb D, Giovanella L, Treglia G. PET imaging in ectopic Cushing's syndrome: a systematic review. Endocrine. 2015;50(2):297-305. doi:10.1007/s12020-015-0689-4. Review.
6. Stratakis CA. Diagnosis and clinical genetics of Cushing syndrome in pediatrics. Endocrinol Metab Clin North Am. 2016;45(2):311-28. doi: 10.1016/j.ecl.2016.01.006. Review.
7. Sulentic P, Morris DG, Grossman A. Cushing's Disease. 2014 Aug 18. In: DeGroot LJ, Chrousos G, Dungan K, Feingold KR, Grossman A, Hershman JM, Koch C, Korbonits M, McLachlan R, New M, Purnell J, Rebar R, Singer F, Vinik A (Eds). Endotext [Internet]. South Dartmouth (MA): MDText.com, Inc.; 2000. Available from *http://www.ncbi.nlm.nih.gov/books/NBK279088/PubMed PMID: 25905314.*
8. Tirosh A, Lodish MB, Papadakis GZ, Lyssikatos C, Belyavskaya E, Stratakis CA. Diurnal plasma cortisol measurements utility in differentiating various etiologies of endogenous Cushing syndrome. Horm Metab Res. 2016;48(10):677-81.

CHAPTER

3

Approach to Hyperprolactinemia

Chitra S

CASE 1

A 29-year-old lady comes to the hospital for complaints of oligomenorrhea for past 3 years. She attained menarche at 14 years and has had regular cycles since then. Over the last three years, she has gained 8–9 kilos of weight gradually. She has no complaints suggestive of galactorrhea, hot flashes or symptoms suggestive of thyroid dysfunction. She has been married for 3 years and wants to plan a pregnancy soon. Her last menstrual period was 15 days ago. She suffers from dyspepsia for which she uses pantoprazole and domperidone tablets 4–5 times a week. Her family has a history of thyroid dysfunction.

On examination, she has a body mass index of 28.5 kg/m^2. On general examination, she has grade 2 goiter, acanthosis, modified Ferriman–Gallwey score of 12/36 and expressive galactorrhea unnoticed before. Clinical examination is not suggestive of any other illness like hypothyroidism or thyrotoxicosis, Cushing's syndrome or acromegaly. Confrontation test is normal. Skin and ankle jerk normal.

Galactorrhea may be overlooked unless actively elicited.

Laboratory Examination Reveals

Thyroid-stimulating hormone (TSH) 2.5 micro IU/L. Total T4 10 µg/dL, prolactin 160 ng/mL, urine pregnancy test negative. Ultrasound pelvis shows ovarian volume 12 cm^3 with numerous cysts in both ovaries peripherally.

A diagnosis of hyperprolactinemia, probably drug induced is made.

Q. 1 How is hyperprolactinemia diagnosed?

Ans. A single sample of prolactin (but not after prolonged fasting or immediately after meals) is drawn without excessive venipuncture stress and prolactin levels assayed. A level greater than the upper limit of normal confirms the diagnosis. Since there are many causes of hyperprolactinemia, it might be prudent to rule out pregnancy, hypothyroidism, medication use and chronic renal failure before assay. It is also important to avoid coitus or nipple stimulation in the last 72 hours before testing. When initial PRL values are not diagnostic (for example, above the normal laboratory range, but not high enough to clearly indicate a prolactinoma), sampling should be repeated on another day obtaining 2–4 samples separated by at least 15–20 min, to avoid the effect of pulsatile secretion.

Q. 2 What are the most common causes of hyperprolactinemia?

Ans. The causes of hyperprolactinemia are many ranging from physiological causes such as exposure to pregnancy, stress exposure to drugs such as antipsychotics, antidepressants, dopamine antagonists like domperidone and oral contraceptive pills. Pituitary stalk compression due to any cause can cause hyperprolactinemia. Prolactinomas are important causes of hyperprolactinemia. Lastly chronic renal failure, polycystic ovary syndrome and hypothyroidism can also be causes of hyperprolactinemia.

Physiological
- Coitus
- Exercise
- Lactation
- Pregnancy
- Stress

Pharmacological
- Anesthetics
- Anticonvulsant
- Antidepressants
- Antihistamines (H_2)
- Antihypertensives
- Cholinergic agonists
- Dopamine receptor blockers
- Dopamine synthesis inhibitor
- Estrogens: oral contraceptives; oral contraceptive withdrawal
- Neuroleptics/antipsychotics
- Neuropeptides
- Opiates and opiate antagonists

Pathological

Hypothalamic-pituitary stalk damage
- Granulomas
- Infiltrations
- Irradiation
- Rathke's cyst
- *Trauma:* Pituitary stalk section, suprasellar surgery
- *Tumors:* Craniopharyngioma, germinoma, hypothalamic metastases, meningioma, suprasellar pituitary mass extension

Pituitary
- Acromegaly
- Idiopathic
- Lymphocytic hypophysitis or parasellar mass
- Macroadenoma (compressive)
- Macroprolactinemia
- Plurihormonal adenoma
- Prolactinoma
- Surgery
- Trauma

Systemic disorders
- Chest—neurogenic chest wall trauma, surgery, herpes zoster
- Chronic renal failure
- Cirrhosis
- Cranial radiation
- Epileptic seizures
- Polycystic ovarian disease

Ref Diagnosis and treatment of hyperprolactinemia. Endocrine Society Clinical practice guideline. JCEM

Q. 3 How is the case 1 patient managed?

Ans. Hyperprolactinemia due to any cause can present with menstrual irregularities with galactorrhea. Most drug induced hyperprolactinemia are in the range of 25–100 ng/mL although dopamine antagonists like risperidone, metoclopramide can cause elevations up to 200 ng/mL. The patient is asked to stop the medications and repeat the assay. Caution must be exercised if the drug involved is antipsychotic medication before stopping. The repeat prolactin in our patient is 130 ng/mL.

As the prolactin levels do not normalize after discontinuation of the drug, magnetic resonance imaging of the hypothalamic pituitary region with dynamic contrast is obtained which reveals a 9 mm microadenoma in the anterior pituitary. A revised diagnosis of microprolactinoma is made.

> Acromegaly can rarely be a cause of galactorrhea with patients with normal prolactin levels.

> Numerous drugs available over-the-counter can increase prolactin levels. A detailed history always helps.

Q. 4 What are the goals of treatment of microprolactinoma?

Ans. The goals of treatment are to normalize gonadal function and restore fertility. Most microadenomas do not increase in size hence suppression of tumor growth is not a treatment goal. In fact asymptomatic patient with micro-prolactinoma can be left untreated and monitored.

Q. 5 What is the first line of management of prolactinomas?

Ans. Dopamine agonist therapy is recommended as first line therapy to lower prolactin levels, decrease tumor size, and restore gonadal function for patients harboring symptomatic prolactin-secreting microadenomas. It is also important to note that microadenomas rarely grow and asymptomatic patients with microadenoma may not need treatment.

Q. 6 How do dopamine agonists work in prolactinomas?

Ans. Dopamine agonists inhibit hormone secretion and reduce cell volume indirectly in an early phase; second, they reduce size of prolactinoma by inhibition of gene transcription and prolactin synthesis and at a later stage, by inducing perivascular fibrosis and cell necrosis.

Q. 7 Why is cabergoline preferred over the other dopamine agonists?

Ans. Cabergoline is recommended in preference to other dopamine agonists because of its longer half-life, higher efficacy in normalizing prolactin levels and tumor shrinkage and better tolerance by patients. Cabergoline is used at doses of 0.125–1 mg/week taken on two days a week. In a placebo-controlled study, cabergoline treatment (0.125–1.0 mg twice weekly) for 12–24 months in patients harboring prolactin-secreting microadenomas resulted in normalization of prolactin levels in 95% of patients. Cabergoline restored menses in 82% of women with amenorrhea.

Our patient is started on cabergoline 0.125 mg twice weekly.

Q. 8 What are the side effects of dopamine agonist agents?

Ans. Nausea occurs in up to 50% of patients. Nasal stuffiness, depression, and digital vasospasm occur, the latter more frequently with higher doses. Postural hypotension, exacerbation of pre-existing psychosis and rarely serious side effects like hepatic dysfunction, cardiac arrhythmia, retroperitoneal fibrosis, pleural effusions have been described. There have been concerns regarding ergot containing dopamine agonists with serotonergic properties (bromocriptine and cabergoline) being associated with a risk for heart valve regurgitation when used in Parkinson's disease in much higher doses and longer duration than hyperprolactinemia. There is no conclusive evidence for such an association at the low doses used for hyperprolactinemia.

Q. 9 How do you initiate dopamine agonists to minimize complications and ensure compliance?

Ans. Usual starting doses are 1.25 mg bromocriptine (daily), or 0.25 mg cabergoline (weekly). Doses of medication are either increased gradually as tolerated, or decreased depending on tolerability, and therapy should begin with a small dose taken with food before bedtime. Patients should initially avoid activities that cause peripheral vasodilatation (e.g. hot baths), to decrease the risk of postural hypotension. Substitution of one medication with another may be beneficial. Intravaginal bromocriptine administration has been used to alleviate adverse gastrointestinal events.

Q. 10 How do you monitor the patient after starting dopamine agonist therapy?

Ans. Patient is monitored clinically for improvements in symptoms and any side effects. Serum prolactin is measured serially. MR imaging can be repeated after normalization of prolactin to document tumor shrinkage.

Q. 11 How long should our patient wait before planning a pregnancy?

Ans. Fertility might be restored even before regular cycles are restored. Hence, it is important to recommend barrier contraception along with the initiation of dopamine agonist therapy. It is recommended that menstrual periods be allowed to occur naturally for a period of time (3–4 months), long enough to predict that a missed period might be a result of pregnancy.

Q. 12 Which dopamine agonist agent is preferred while planning conception?

Ans. The incidence of abortions, ectopic pregnancies or congenital malformations is no higher in infants born to mothers who conceived while taking bromocriptine than that in the general population. Similar results have been reported with women who have taken cabergoline before and during pregnancy. Thus, both the dopamine agonists are considered safe in the period prior to and during pregnancy although the number of pregnancies studied using cabergoline are smaller than bromocriptine.

Q. 13 Should we continue dopamine agonist after conception in our patient with microadenoma?

Ans. Microadenomas have a lesser chance of symptomatic tumor enlargement during pregnancy. Although dopamine agonists especially bromocriptine has been used in pregnancy and no adverse fetal effects have been documented, it is prudent to eliminate risk of fetal exposure to any drug once conception occurs. Hence, in our patient with microadenoma, it is recommended that the dopamine agonist be stopped once the pregnancy test is positive.

Q. 14 How does one follow-up our patient with microprolactinoma during pregnancy?

Ans. There is no role of monitoring serum prolactin serially in pregnancy as during normal pregnancy, serum prolactin levels increase 10 folds. Hence, following up on serial prolactin may not represent tumor growth. Patients are followed by purely based on symptoms such as severe headache or visual field compromise.

Q. 15 Would the recommendation be any different if it was a patient with macroadenoma wishing for a pregnancy?

Ans. In the case of a macroadenoma, the risk of symptomatic tumor enlargement during pregnancy is as high as 31%. Thus, the decision to stop treatment at diagnosis of pregnancy is not unanimous. There are two equally rational things that could be done, one stop treatment and monitor for symptoms and visual field testing every trimester and restart treatment if new changes occur. This option is preferred in patients who have macroadenoma confined to the sella and macroadenoma without visual compromise. The second is to continue treatment during pregnancy, an option preferred in patients who had visual complaints at diagnosis.

Q. 16 Can our patient breastfeed?

Ans. Women wishing to breastfeed their infants should not be given dopamine agonists because the resulting decrease in serum PRL levels will impair lactation. There is no data to suggest that breastfeeding leads to an increase in tumor size.

Q. 17 Will our patient need dopamine agonist therapy after delivery and breastfeeding?

Ans. Pregnancy may ameliorate antepartum hyperprolactinemia completely. Hence, it is best to wait and reassess if symptoms of amenorrhea and/or oligoamenorrhea recur before evaluating for hyperprolactinemia.

Q. 18 If the above discussed patient did not desire to conceive, how long will she be on dopamine agonist therapy?

Ans. The minimal length of dopamine agonist therapy should be 1 year. Some patients may remain in long-term remission after a period of dopamine agonist treatment. If a patient has normal. PRL levels after therapy with dopamine agonists for at least 3 years and the tumor volume is markedly reduced, an attempt at tapering of drugs may be initiated. Patients need to be followed to detect recurrence of hyperprolactinemia and tumor enlargement so that treatment can be promptly resumed.

CASE 2

A friend of our patient who has regular cycles and no galactorrhea, after hearing about our patient's condition, goes in for a prolactin assay. She is not on any drugs and is euthyroid. On examination, there is no galactorrhea. Her prolactin levels are 74 ng/mL. Polyethylene glycol precipitation revealed that 80% of prolactin was macroprolactin.

Q. 1 What is macroprolactin? When should one check for it?

Ans. Normally 85% of circulating prolactin is monomeric (23.5 kDa). The remaining 15% is made of a covalently bound dimer, "big prolactin," and a much larger polymeric form, "big big prolactin." The term macroprolactinemia denotes the situation in which a preponderance of the circulating prolactin consists of these larger molecules. Macroprolactin are less bioactive, and macroprolactinemia should be suspected when typical symptoms of hyperprolactinemia are absent.

> Macroprolactin should be tested in patients with hyperprolactinemia who are asymptomatic.

CASE 3

A 27-year-old man present with complaints of loss of libido and erectile dysfunction since a year. On questioning, he gives history of headache, dull aching, global, not associated with nausea or vomiting, usually relieved by painkillers, present on 5 days a week. He has also noticed that sometimes he bumped into objects on his sides while walking. He has also noticed constipation and weight gain.

On examination, he is 160 cm tall with a BMI 25 kg/m^2. Blood pressure 110/70 mm of Hg, no postural drop. Confrontation test reveals bilateral temporal hemianopia. Testicular volume 15 mL soft bilateral. No galactorrhea is elicited. Ankle jerks delayed.

Laboratory investigations are as follows:

Hemoglobin 10.5 g/dL, normocytic normochromic anemia.

Testosterone 100 ng/dL, LH 0.01 IU/L, FSH 0.01 IU/L, TSH 2 microIU/L, free T4 0.68 ng/dL. Cortisol 2.8 μg/dL. Prolactin 47 ng/mL from one lab and 1780 ng/mL from another lab. Automated perimetry reveal bitemporal hemianopia. Magnetic resonance imaging of the hypothalamic pituitary region reveals 2.4 cm tall, pituitary mass with suprasellar extension with compression of the optic chiasm without parasellar extension.

A diagnosis of pituitary macroadenoma probably macroprolactinoma with hypopituitarism is made.

Q. 1 Why is there a discrepancy in the prolactin assay from the laboratory?

Ans. The probable reason for the discrepancy is the hook effect, an assay artifact that may be seen when high serum prolactin concentrations saturate antibodies in the two-site immunoassay.

The presence of excess amounts of the prolactin in the unbound state, binds to the signaling antibody alone and is washed out without binding to the capture antibody, leading to a false low result. This can be averted by either diluting the sample or by allowing a washout after adding the serum to remove excess unbound prolactin before adding signaling antibody.

Many newer assays have higher upper limits of detection, thereby reducing chances of a high dose hook effect.

Thus, when prolactin values are not as high as expected, the assay should be repeated after a 1:100 serum sample dilution to overcome a potential hook effect.

Q. 2 Why is there no galactorrhea despite elevated prolactin levels in this patient?

Ans. Only 35% of men with prolactinomas have galactorrhea as the male mammary tissue is less susceptible to lactogenic effect of hyperprolactinemia. Even in women only 50% have galactorrhea as the lactogenic effect is seen in oestrogen primed mammary tissue. So if the patient has been hypogonadal for a long duration, there may be no galactorrhea.

Q. 3 Could it be that this patient is harboring a nonfunctioning tumor and the elevated prolactin is due to stalk compression?

Ans. Hyperprolactinemia in the presence of an MRI-detected pituitary adenoma is consistent with but not unequivocally diagnostic of a prolactinoma, because any pituitary mass that compresses the pituitary stalk may cause hyperprolactinemia. A therapeutic trial with dopamine agonists for a period of time leading to decrease in prolactin levels serially and shrinkage in tumor size is diagnostic of prolactinoma. All patients with a macroadenoma with elevated prolactin warrant a treatment course with dopamine agonist.

Q. 4 Why is our patient anemic?

Ans. Anemia is common (40%) in patients with macroprolactinoma and shows association with hypogonadism and tumor size and improves following treatment that normalizes prolactin and increases testosterone.

Q. 5 Is the visual field defect not an urgent indication for surgery?

Ans. Dopamine agonists usually restore visual function to an extent similar to that produced by surgical decompression of the chiasm in macroprolactinoma patients. Therefore, patients with macroprolactinomas who have visual field defects are no longer considered to be neurosurgical emergencies.

Q. 6 How is the hypopituitarism managed in this patient?

Ans. Patients with macroprolactinomas (>10 mm in diameter) and hypopituitarism should receive standard hormone replacement therapy as any other patient with one exception. Initiation of growth hormone (GH) and gonadal steroid replacement should be delayed until after normoprolactinemia and/or tumor shrinkage are achieved, given that both GH and gonadal steroid deficiencies can be restored by normalization of prolactin levels compared with other deficiencies of the pituitary axis.

Q. 7 Is the initiating dose of cabergoline higher in macroprolactinoma as compared to microprolactinoma considering there is an urgent need to decompress in view of the visual compromise?

Ans. The initiating dose of cabergoline, counter intuitively is lower for macroprolactinoma with doses of 0.25 mg/week to avoid too rapid shrinkage of tumor which might precipitate intratumoral hemorrhage necessitating surgical decompression or CSF rhinorrhea.

Q. 8 How will this patient be monitored after initiation of therapy?

Ans. The patient is monitored as a patient with microadenoma but will need visual field assessment to monitor recovery and MR imaging at 3–4 months to document tumor shrinkage.

Q. 9 Will the patient be able to be stop dopamine agonists?

Ans. If the PRL level has been normal for at least 2 years and the size of the tumor decreased by more than 50%, an attempt to decrease the dose of the dopamine agonist can be made, because at this stage low doses are likely to maintain stable PRL levels and tumor size.

However, in patients with macroadenomas cessation of therapy may lead to tumor expansion and recurrence of hyperprolactinemia. Hence, close follow-up is necessary when the drug is tapered or withdrawn in patients with macroprolactinomas.

Q. 10 What are the treatment options available to the patient is unable to tolerate or is unresponsive to dopamine agonists?

Ans. The first step is to increase dose of dopamine agonists. Cabergoline is found to be effective in patients resistant to bromocriptine. Trans-sphenoidal surgery is an option for patient who are symptomatic and are unresponsive to dopamine agonists. For patients who fail surgical treatment, radiation therapy is an option although the lag period can run into years to see the effects.

SUGGESTED READING

1. Caloa A, Savanstano S. Medical treatment of prolactinomas. Nat Rev Endocrinol. 2011;7:267-78.
2. Guidelines of the Pituitary Society for the diagnosis and management of prolactinomas. Clinical Endocrinology. 2006;65:265-73.
3. Melmed S, Kleinberg D. Pituitary Masses and Tumours. Chap 9 Williams Textbook of Endocrinology.
4. Shimon I, Benbassat C, Tzvetov G, Grozinsky-Glasberg S. Anemia in a cohort of men with macroprolactinomas: increase in hemoglobin levels follows prolactin suppression. Pituitary. 2011;14(1):11-5
5. Webster J, Piscitelli G, Polli A, Ferrari CI, Ismail I, Scanlon MF. a comparison of cabergoline and bromocriptine in the treatment of hyperprolactinemic amenorrhoea. Cabergoline Comparative Study Group. New England Journal of Medicine. 1994; 331:904-9.

CHAPTER

4

Pseudo- and Iatrogenic Cushing's Syndrome

Chitra S, Prashant Kaduskar

CASE 1

A 28-year-old lady presents with complaints of fatigue, inability to climb stairs, since the last two years. She is irritable and has bouts of crying and has stopped pursuing her job as a teacher and prefers to stay at home. She has been found to have hyperglycemia requiring treatment for the same time. Most of her complaints started about 2 years ago when she was put on herbal supplements to increase her appetite and body weight.

On examination, she is conscious, appears lost in thought, has thin skin on the dorsum of her hand, purple-colored striae on her abdomen and calves measuring around 1 cm in width. She has patches of red bruises on her inner arms. Her waist circumference is 96 cm and blood pressure is 150/90 mm Hg. She has proximal myopathy of both upper and lower limbs. She has no hirsutism or increased pigmentation.

A clinical diagnosis of Cushing's syndrome is made. She is asked to stop her herbal supplements. An 8 am cortisol assay is done which reveals cortisol of <0.1 µg/dL.

A diagnosis of exogenous Cushing's syndrome is made.

Q. 1 What is Cushing's syndrome?

Ans. It is a syndrome characterized by signs and symptoms associated with prolonged exposure to inappropriately high levels of plasma glucocorticoids. The glucocorticoids can be exogenous or endogenous. Cushing's syndrome due to exogenous glucocorticoids is called Iatrogenic Cushing's syndrome. Endogenous glucocorticoids can be ACTH dependent or ACTH independent. Iatrogenic Cushing's is the most common form of Cushing's syndrome.

> Iatrogenic Cushing's is the most common cause of Cushing's syndrome.

Q. 2 What are the features of iatrogenic Cushing's syndrome?

Ans. Although most clinical manifestations overlap with endogenous Cushing's syndrome, some features can be strikingly different in iatrogenic Cushing's syndrome. The classical symptoms of weight gain, obesity, dorsocervical and supraclavicular fat pads, facial plethora, easy bruising; thin skin, striae, myopathy, and muscle weakness (particularly proximal muscles) are seen in both. Poor wound healing and susceptibility to infection is common. Psychological adverse effects like depression and psychosis can be severe. Metabolic complications like hypertension, hyperglycemia and dyslipidemia also occur.

Some manifestations of glucocorticoid excess occur relatively quickly. Psychiatric effects, insomnia, and increased appetite can occur within hours. Generally, a cushingoid appearance takes weeks or even months to develop, as does development of osteoporosis.

- All the features of endogenous Cushing's can be present in iatrogenic Cushing's syndrome.
- Psychological effects are acute and can be quite severe.

Q. 3 Are there any differences in symptoms of iatrogenic and endogenous Cushing's features?

Ans. There are few clinical features which are more common and some features which are less common in iatrogenic Cushing's.

Hypertension though common in iatrogenic Cushing's, these patients may have relatively less hypertension and hypokalemia compared with patients who have spontaneous Cushing's syndrome depending on the mineralocorticoid activity of the steroid they are taking.

Patients with iatrogenic Cushing's syndrome are less likely to have significant increases in androgens, and therefore they have less hirsutism and other virilizing features than those who have spontaneous disease.

There is increased incidence of glaucoma and other ocular disease such as posterior subcapsular cataracts in these patients.

Avascular necrosis is more common in iatrogenic than in spontaneous Cushing's syndrome.

Osteoporosis is a common and severe adverse effect of glucocorticoid excess and one of the major limitations to long-term glucocorticoid therapy. A significant number of patients on long-term steroid therapy will have at least some loss of bone density. Oral and inhaled corticosteroid uses are associated with increased bone fractures. The bone loss caused by glucocorticoids tends to be in trabecular bone as opposed to cortical bone. Therefore, most loss is in the vertebrae and ribs of the axial skeleton.

- Hypertension, hypokalemia, androgenic features like hirsutism and oligoamenorrhea are less common in iatrogenic Cushing's syndrome.
- Certain features such as posterior subcapsular cataract, glaucoma, avascular necrosis of femur osteoporosis and pancreatitis are more common in iatrogenic Cushing's syndrome than endogenous Cushing's syndrome.

Q. 4 What are the factors that play a role in the development of iatrogenic Cushing's syndrome?

Ans. Multiple factors decide the effects of steroids and hence the development of iatrogenic Cushing's syndrome. Steroids are available in many different preparations and have different modes of delivery. Although the use of topical, intra-articular, or aerosol therapy has the advantage of allowing more targeted therapy and therefore theoretically fewer systemic adverse effects, every mode of steroid treatment can cause Cushing's features.

Relevant properties of the steroids themselves include the formulation used, pharmacokinetics, affinity for the glucocorticoid receptor, biologic potency, and duration of action.

Pharmacokinetic factors include binding affinities to cortisol-binding globulin (CBG) and other plasma proteins, metabolic inactivation, and plasma half-life. Most synthetic glucocorticoids do not have significant binding to CBG and bind instead to albumin or circulate as free steroid. In contrast, synthetic glucocorticoids have a much higher affinity for the glucocorticoid receptor than cortisol itself. However, these are theoretical considerations and relative estimate of glucocorticoid activity and hence development of Cushing's features cannot be predicted.

Specific modes of delivery have different effects. Oral steroid use is most common form likely to cause Cushing's features. Topical steroids do get systemically absorbed and this may further be enhanced by breakdown of skin integrity. Inhaled glucocorticoids initially thought to be safe do have side effects particularly bone, ocular, and skin manifestations. Cushing's syndrome has been reported in patients taking relatively high doses of intra-articular glucocorticoids. Pediatric cases of intra-articular and intradermal steroid injections causing Cushing's syndrome have been reported.

> The minimum dose of steroid required for development of Cushing's syndrome is the equivalent of prednisolone in dose of 7.5 mg for 3 months.

CASE 2

A 48-year-old lady has been referred from her primary physician to rule out Cushing's disease. She has been suffering with bronchial asthma for 20 years, with acute exacerbations at least 3 times/year requiring hospital admissions. She is on inhaled steroids everyday with use of oral steroids for 1–2 weeks at least 4–6 times/year. She is also diagnosed to have diabetes and hypertension for 5 years and is on treatment. She had sustained fracture of the left wrist following a trivial fall a year ago. On examination, she has central obesity, abdominal striae, thin skin and hypertension. Her primary physician ordered for an 8 am cortisol which showed 28 μg/dL.

After receiving the patient, it is revealed that the patient was continuing to use prednisolone 10 mg/day without disclosing to her doctor. She is educated about being off all medications and a repeat 8 am cortisol is ordered which is 2 μg/dL this time suggesting exogenous cortisol use.

Q. 1 How is a diagnosis of exogenous Cushing's syndrome made?

Ans. An 8 am cortisol assay if found suppressed (generally accepted as <5 μg/dL), endogenous hypercortisolism can be ruled out and a diagnosis of exogenous Cushing's syndrome can be made. It is important to remember that most synthetic steroid preparations have assay interference with cortisol, hence, if a patient is continuing to take the steroid while being tested, the report may be falsely normal or high. Close monitoring, preferably after admission to exclude surreptitious use of steroid (as in case 2) is necessary.

Q. 2 What are the factors to be considered while withdrawing steroids?

Ans. The discontinuation of steroid therapy can present a significant clinical challenge and following three factors need to be considered while withdrawing steroids—(1) the possibility of suppression of the hypothalamic–pituitary–adrenal (HPA) axis and resulting secondary adrenal insufficiency, (2) the possibility of worsening of the underlying disease for which steroid therapy was initiated, and (3) a phenomenon, sometimes called the steroid withdrawal syndrome, in which some patients encounter difficulty, and even significant symptoms, discontinuing or decreasing steroid doses despite having demonstrably normal HPA axes.

Q. 3 How to taper steroids in patients on long-term steroids with iatrogenic Cushing's?

Ans. Patients on long-term steroid therapy should be offered withdrawal of steroid therapy in following way.

There is a paucity of randomized trials which have looked at the best possible method of tapering steroids. Most are based on regimens that have been followed.

Any patient with steroid use for less than 3 weeks can be stopped without tapering.

Any patient on prednisolone >5 mg for >3 weeks undergoes tapering by 2.5 mg every 3–4 days till the patient is brought down to 5 mg/day. Once the patient is on 5 mg/day, the patient is shifted to the equivalent dose of hydrocortisone 20 mg as it has a shorter half-life and is easier to taper down (as compared to prednisolone). Hydrocortisone is then tapered at the rate of 2.5 mg/1–2 weeks to reach hydrocortisone 10 mg/day in the morning. At this point, the patient is maintained on hydrocortisone 10 mg/day for 2–3 months allowing the axis sufficient time to recover. At the end of 3 months, a synacthen stimulation test can be done to decide if the patient can go off steroids if they have a cortisol value >18 μg/dL. Another way of assessing recovery is doing an 8 am cortisol after omitting the hydrocortisone dose for the day. If the cortisol level >10 μg/dL steroids can be withdrawn with advice for stress dose when infections occur. Most often steroid withdrawal is far from the smooth tapering regimens we design. Conditions for which they were on steroids in the first place may flare up requiring increase in steroid dose. Second, most patients on steroids for a long time, are used to the euphoric sense of well-being they provide and tend to take a step or two back in the tapering program without informing the clinician (Table 4.1).

TABLE 4.1 Tapering schedule of steroids

Prednisolone dose	*Duration of therapy*		
mg/d	*<3 weeks*		*>3 weeks*
7.5 mg	Can stop		↓ rapidly (2.5 mg q3–4d) then
5.0 mg	Can stop	↓ 1 mg q2–4 week then	OR convert 5 mg pred to HC 20 mg, then ↓ 2.5 mg/week to 10 mg/day then
<5.0 mg	Can stop	↓ 1 mg q2–4 week	After 2–3 months at hydrocortisone 10 mg/d, administer SST/ITT : *Pass:* Withdraw *Fail:* Continue

In patients taking prednisolone 5–7.5 mg/d or equivalent corticosteroid, SST 12–24 hours after omitted dose of steroid to decide sudden or gradual withdrawal.

Q. 4 How to manage osteoporosis in iatrogenic Cushing's syndrome?

Ans. According to the recommendations of the American College of Rheumatology (ACR) from 2010, the glucocorticoid dose and the duration of therapy should be reduced to a minimum, which is clinically effective in specific diseases, such as rheumatoid arthritis, asthma or others. The glucocorticoid dose reduction and shortening therapy duration minimizes the risk of fractures.

Similar to the general recommendations for osteoporosis treatment, lifestyle modifications, consisting of regular physical activity including exercises with own body weight, fall prevention, smoking cessation, limiting alcohol, compensation of calcium deficiency to a total intake of 1200–1500 mg/day and control of vitamin D3 alteration of 25-hydroxyvitamin D3 concentration are also very important. A recommended preventive dose of vitamin D3 is 800–1000 IU per day.

Monitoring patient's height and Bone Mineral Density (BMD) is also essential in glucocorticoid therapy. The ACR recommends radiological or morphometric assessment of the spine in patients receiving 5 mg or more of prednisolone daily. Before starting treatment, the assessment of global fracture risk based on the presence of other known coexisting risk factors beyond steroids, such as low BMI, parental hip fracture, current smoking, consumption of more than 3 units of alcohol a day and a significant decrease in BMD should also be considered.

American College of Rheumatology recommendations distinguish two groups of patients: Premenopausal women and men less than 50 years of age and postmenopausal women and men over 50 years of age. In the former group as there are no adequate studies and guidelines, individual approach is recommended. For patients with osteoporotic fractures receiving ≥5 mg prednisolone or equivalent for more than a month, it is recommended to start treatment with bisphosphonates of proven effectiveness in glucocorticoid-induced osteoporosis, such as alendronate or risedronate, and if steroid dose is ≥7.5 mg, zoledronic acid should also be considered. If treatment with glucocorticoids is continued for a period of 3 months then, regardless of the dose, the patient should receive one of four treatment options: alendronate, risedronate, zoledronate or teriparatide.

The patients in the second group of the ACR recommendations should be divided into three subgroups, depending on the established global fracture risk, calculated on the basis of well proven algorithms, such as FRAX (low, medium or high fracture risk). Among patients with low or medium fracture risk, it is recommended to start therapy with alendronate, risedronate or zoledronate, if steroid administration exceeds 3 months and daily dose is ≥7.5 mg of prednisolone or equivalent. In patients with an average risk of fracture, it is advisable to administer alendronate and risedronate if steroid daily dose is <7.5 mg of prednisolone or equivalent and the patient has been treated for ≥3 months. Patients with high fracture risk should receive one out of the following three drugs: alendronate, risedronate or zoledronate, if they use steroids in a dose of <5 mg/day, even for <1 month, and when they receive >5 mg glucocorticoids per day, teriparatide should be considered.

Q. 5 How should patients with glucocorticoid-induced osteoporosis be monitored?

Ans. Although BMD assessment is not the best modality to quantify micro-architectural damage caused by steroids, they still remain the main monitoring parameter in glucocorticoid induced osteoporosis, owing to a lack of a better feasible mode. The DXA scans should be performed at 1–2 years interval. In addition, at each visit the patient should have assessed the risk of falls, height, medication compliance, and if required, the concentration of 25-hydroxyvitamin D3 and an X-ray of the spine.

CASE 3

A 47-year-old lady with complaints of decreased ability to sleep has been admitted under the department of psychiatry and found to have depression with generalized anxiety disorder. She has also been diagnosed with diabetes and hypertension for 4 years for which she is on metformin 2 g/day with glimepiride 4 mg/day and amlodipine 10 mg/day. She has oligoamenorrhea for many years and has cycles only after taking medroxyprogesterone acetate for 5 days. On examination, her BMI is 31 kg/m^2, has waist circumference of 102 cm, acanthosis nigricans, no striae or bruising. Blood pressure of 140/90 mm Hg. Her psychiatry consultant wants to rule out Cushing's syndrome as a cause of the depression and metabolic features.

What would you do next?

Q. 1 What is pseudo-Cushing's syndrome?

Ans. Pseudo-Cushing's states can be defined as a condition where some or all of the clinical features of Cushing's syndrome with some evidence of hyper-cortisolism. Resolution of the underlying primary condition leads to disappea-rance of the signs and symptoms of Cushing's syndrome.

Q. 2 What is the importance of diagnosing pseudo-Cushing's state?

Ans. It is quite important to determine if the patient has Cushing's syndrome or a pseudo-Cushing's state in a time- and cost-effective manner, because if a patient with a pseudo-Cushing's state is misdiagnosed as having Cushing's syndrome, that patient could undergo needless testing and unnecessary surgery. On the other hand, it is important to identify Cushing's syndrome accurately as it is a condition with increased mortality and morbidity.

Q. 3 What are the causes of pseudo-Cushing's syndrome?

Ans.

- *Some clinical features of Cushing's syndrome may be present:*[8]
  - Pregnancy
  - Depression and other psychiatric conditions
  - Alcohol dependence
  - Glucocorticoid resistance
  - Morbid obesity
  - Poorly controlled diabetes mellitus
- *Unlikely to have any clinical features of Cushing's syndrome:*
  - Physical stress (hospitalization, surgery, pain)
  - Malnutrition, anorexia nervosa
  - Intense chronic exercise
  - Hypothalamic amenorrhea
  - Cortisol-blinding globulin excess (increased serum but not urine cortisol).

Q. 4 What is the pathogenesis of pseudo-Cushing's syndrome?

Ans. Many of the conditions mentioned above have underlying defect in HPA axis or other physiological mechanism which leads to pseudo-Cushing's state.

Depression: It is hypothesized that endogenous CRH is elevated in depression. The adrenal glands would then hypertrophy leading to the increased response of cortisol to ACTH. Cortisol feedback to the corticotroph would remain present, although also blunted. Most of these changes are reversible after recovery from depression.

Alcoholism: There is a hypersecretion of CRH in chronic alcohol abuse and chronic liver disease. Also, in alcoholism, there appears to be impaired binding of cortisol to cortisol-binding globulin (CBG), leading to elevated levels of free cortisol. Another possible explanation for pseudo-Cushing's syndrome in patients with alcohol abuse is impaired hepatic metabolism of cortisol. Lastly, AVP levels are elevated in patients with decompensated liver disease which may stimulate cortisol secretion.

Obesity: In obesity, there is an activation of HPA axis, probably attributed to increased metabolism of cortisol.

The other causes of pseudo-Cushing's are less likely to have clinical features of Cushing's syndrome but only have biochemical hypercortisolism.

Q. 5 What are the tests available for differentiating pseudo-Cushing's from Cushing's syndrome?

Ans. The tests that are used to rule out pseudo–Cushing's syndrome are essentially screening tests for Cushing's syndrome with a relatively greater specificity for identifying Cushing's syndrome.

- *Low-dose dexamethasone test:* In conditions where the probability of pseudo–Cushing's disease is high, LDDST may be an optimal screening test as it has greater specificity as compared to overnight dexamethasone test or 24 hours urine cortisol levels.

  In the LDDST, dexamethasone (0.5 mg) is given every 6 hours for eight doses and the serum cortisol assessed after that. It is important to acknowledge that conditions that alter cortisol-binding globulin levels can interfere with the test results as are ingestion of drugs which alter dexamethasone metabolism. With a cut-off value of 1.8 μg/dL, the sensitivity ranges from 90% to 95%. Not all studies that have explored LDDST have reported similar results, but of the tests available, LDDST is preferred first line test.
- *Midnight serum cortisol:* Midnight serum cortisol value >7.5 ug/dL is diagnostic of Cushing's syndrome. In a study by Papanicolaou, et al. using this cut-off correctly identified 225/234 patients with Cushing's syndrome, while a value less than this cut-off was found in all 23 patients with pseudo-Cushing's states. Thus, the specificity was 100% and the sensitivity was 96%.

  Where there is a low clinical index of suspicion, such as in simple obesity, but lack of suppression on dexamethasone testing and mildly elevated UFC, a sleeping midnight serum cortisol less than 1.8 μg/dL effectively excludes Cushing's syndrome at the time of assessment.
- *Midnight salivary cortisol:* One study examined 11 PM salivary cortisol in 39 patients with proven Cushing's syndrome. The average 11 PM salivary cortisol was 20 times higher in the patients with Cushing's syndrome than the other two groups. Using a cut-off of 3.6 nmol/L (0.13 μg/dL), 36/39 patients with Cushing's syndrome had an elevated value, while 38/39 of the normal volunteers had values less than the cut-off. The sensitivity and specificity of this test was 92% and 96%, respectively. The ability to assay cortisol from saliva is not widely available in India.
- *Dexamethasone-CRH test:* The dexamethasone test takes advantage of the fact that in patients with Cushing's syndrome, dexamethasone ineffectively suppresses the production of pituitary ACTH. CRH stimulates the pituitary to secrete ACTH which leads to an increase in cortisol levels. Patients with Cushing's syndrome have a larger increase in plasma ACTH and cortisol levels than in normal individuals or those patients with pseudo-Cushing's states after injection of CRH.

  In one study 39 patients with Cushing's syndrome and 19 patients with pseudo-Cushing's state underwent the combined test. Patients received dexamethasone (0.5 mg) 4 times a day for 2 days starting at 12 noon (last dose at 6 am). At 8 am on the day of the last dose, the patients received intravenous ovine CRH (1 μg/kg) and cortisol and ACTH were measured at various times.

A plasma cortisol greater than 1.4 µg/dL (38 nmol/L) measured 15 minutes after the CRH injection correctly identified all patients with Cushing's syndrome, while a value less than 1.4 µg/dL identified all patients with pseudo-Cushing's states (100% sensitivity and specificity). Of course, CRH is difficult to procure in India.

- *Loperamide test:* Loperamide decreases ACTH and cortisol levels. The opiate agonist is given at a dose of 16 mg at 8:30 AM and 3 samples (basal, 180 and 210 min after drug) are obtained. In 41 patients with confirmed Cushing's syndrome, loperamide did not suppress the cortisol levels below 138 nmol/L (5 µg/dL), while in 104 of 110 patients referred for evaluation of Cushing's syndrome, which was subsequently ruled out, the cortisol value suppressed to less than 138 nmol/L (5 µg/dL) at either 150 or 210 min. This test has not been validated nor routinely used in our clinical setting.

  Other tests that have been used but not recommended are Insulin tolerance test, IL-6 test and desmopressin test.

Q. 6 How is the patient in Case 3 managed?

Ans. As the pretest probability of Cushing's syndrome is low and that of pseudo-Cushing's high, she is subjected to midnight serum cortisol which is 1.4 µg/dL and her LDDST is 0.6 µg/dL. Hence, Cushing's syndrome is ruled out and she is followed up.

Q. 7 What is the treatment of pseudo-Cushing's syndrome?

Ans. The treatment essentially consists of treating the underlying cause. Careful interpretation of relevant screening tests are suggested. Serial follow-up of patients and watchful observation of development of any new features of Cushing's syndrome and retesting when appropriate, are recommended.

SUGGESTED READING

1. Ambrosi B, Bochicchio D, Colombo P, Fadin C, Faglia G. Loperamide to diagnose Cushing's syndrome. J Am Med Assoc. 1993;270:2301-2.
2. Groote Veldman R, Meinders AE. On the mechanism of alcohol-induced pseudo-Cushing's syndrome. Endocr Rev. 1996;17:262-8.
3. Grossman JM, Gordon R, Ranganath VK, Deal C, Caplan L, Chen W, et al. American College of Rheumatology 2010 Recommendations for the Prevention and Treatment of Glucocorticoid-Induced Osteoporosis. Arthritis Care Res (Hoboken). 2010;62: 1515-26.
4. Israel E, Banerjee TR, Fitzmaurice GM, et al. Effects of inhaled glucocorticoids on bone density in premenopausal women. N Engl J Med. 2001;345(13):941-7.
5. Jansen TL, Van Roon EN. Four cases of a secondary Cushingoid state following local triamcinolone acetonide (Kenacort) injection. Neth J Med. 2002;60(3):151-3.
6. Jobling AI, Augusteyn RC. What causes steroid cataracts? A review of steroid-induced posterior subcapsular cataracts. Clin Exp Optom. 2002;85(2):61-75.
7. Kumar S, Singh RJ, Reed AM, et al. Cushing's syndrome after intra-articular and intradermal administration of triamcinolone acetonide in three pediatric patients. Pediatrics. 2004;113(6):1820-4.

8. Laan R, van Reil P, van de Putte L, et al. Low-dose prednisone induces rapid reversible axial bone loss in patients with rheumatoid arthritis. Ann Intern Med. 1993;119(10): 963-8.
9. Lipworth BJ. Systemic adverse effects of inhaled corticosteroid therapy: a systematic review and meta-analysis. Arch Intern Med. 1999;159(9):941-55.
10. Mankin HJ. Nontraumatic necrosis of bone (osteonecrosis). N Engl J Med. 1992;326(22):1473-9.
11. Neiman et al. Guidelines for the diagnosis of Cushing's syndrome. J Clin Endocrinol Metab. 2008;93(5):1526-40.
12. Orth DN, Kovacs WJ. The adrenal cortex. In: Wilson JD (Ed). Williams Textbook of Endocrinology, 9th edn. Philadelphia: WB Saunders Company; 1998. pp. 605-10.
13. S Hopkins RL, Leinung MC. Exogenous Cushing' syndrome and glucocorticoid withdrawal. Endocrinol Metab North Am. 2005;34:371-84.
14. Theodore Friedman. What is Pseudo-Cushing's? Chapter in Adrenal Disorders. Margioris AN, Chrousos GP (Eds).
15. Van Staa T, Leufkens H, Abenhaim L, et al. Use of oral corticosteroids and risk of fractures. J Bone Miner Res. 2000;15:993-1000.
16. Van Staa T, Leufkens H, Cooper C. Use of inhaled corticosteroids and risk of fractures. J Bone Miner Res. 2001;16:581-8.

CHAPTER

5

Approach to a Child with Delayed Puberty

Anu Vishwanath

CASE

A 17-year 3-month-old male presents with concern for short stature. Patient is short, appears well-nourished, has no dysmorphic features, is normotensive, and noted to be prepubertal.

Past medical history: Patient has been well and has not had any chronic illnesses nor has he been on any chronic medications. Parents report that he has always been among the shorter children at school.

Birth history: Patient was born at full term by normal vaginal delivery. His birth weight was 2.5 kg and his birth length is not available.

Developmental history: Parents report normal developmental milestones. No history of delayed dentition.

Diet history: Patient consumes about 1800 kcal/day.

Family history: Patient lives with his parents and younger brother. No reported medical or hormonal disorders in the immediate or extended family.

Social history: Patient is studying in twelfth grade and reported good grades.

Physical examination: Patient is noted to be 147 cm tall (–3.5 SD below mean) and 40 kg (–1.88 SD below mean). No evidence of goiter. Patient is noted to be tanner 1 for pubic hair with tanner 1 prepubertal testicles. Other systemic exam is within normal limits.

Labs

- Normal CBC, electrolytes, S. calcium and phosphorus, renal function, liver function and urinalysis
- AM cortisol noted to be 4.6 μg/dL, stimulated cortisol level 15 μg/dL
- FSH 0.51 mIU/mL, LH 0.10 mIU/mL, Testosterone <2.5 ng/dL

- Prolactin 11.44 ng/mL
- TSH 0.019 mcIU/L (0.6–5.5), fT4 0.6 ng/dL (0.8–1.7)
- Testosterone primed GH stimulation testing with clonidine noting peak GH level below 3 ng/mL.

Q. 1 What are the changes expected to occur during puberty?

Ans.

- Appearance of secondary sexual characteristics
  In girls—appearance of breast bud (thelarche) is usually the first sign of puberty, followed by the appearance of pubic hair (pubarche) 6–12 months later, and accompanied by growth spurt associated with puberty, appearance of axillary hair and, acne
  In boys—the pubertal changes include growth of the testes (≥4 mL in volume or 2.5 cm longitudinal measurement), followed by thinning of the scrotum, pigmentation of the scrotum, growth of the penis, pubarche, acceleration of growth, breaking of voice, appearance of axillary hair, facial hair, acne
- Pubertal growth spurt—In girls, peak height velocity occurs at breast stage II–III and in boys maximal growth rate occurs at genital stage IV–V
- Maturation of reproductive capacity manifested by menarche (which usually occurs about 2–2.5 years after puberty initiation) in females and spermaturia in males.

Premature adrenarche is elevation of DHEAS levels (which is derived from adrenal glands) before the age of 8 years in girls and 9 years in boys and the concurrent presence of signs of androgen action, including adult-type body odor, oily skin and hair and/or pubic hair growth.

Q. 2 When is puberty delayed?

Ans. Delayed puberty is usually defined as the failure to manifest the initial signs of sexual maturation by an age that is more than 2–2.5 SDS (standard deviation score) above the mean for the population (>13 year in girls and 14 year in boys).

- For girls this is usually defined by absence of pubertal development by age 13 years, marked by no appearance of secondary sexual characteristics and no menarche
- For boys, this is usually defined as absence of testicular enlargement by age 14 years.

Primary amenorrhea: No menarche by age 16 years in the presence of secondary sexual characteristics.

Q. 3 What are the causes of delayed puberty ?

Ans. Causes of delayed puberty could be broadly classified as

- Central (hypothalamus/pituitary) causes leading to tertiary or secondary hypogonadotropic hypogonadism
- Peripheral (gonadal) leading to primary hypergonadotropic hypogonadism
- Variants of normal such as constitutional delay of growth and puberty.

Q. 4 What investigations would be indicated in patients presenting with delayed puberty?

Ans. Evaluation of delayed puberty should include a detailed history, thorough physical exam to assess nutritional status, biochemical testing for hormone levels and to look for any systemic diseases, and may entail imaging modalities such as bone age X-ray.

History: Childhood growth patterns and development medical or surgical history to rule out any chronic systemic, autoimmune or endocrine diseases, history of any radiation exposure, any complaints of anosmia, assessment of diet and nutritional status, exercise and activity. History of any prolonged jaundice at birth or recurrent hypoglycemia, seizures should be elicited. Family history of pubertal delay or infertility should be obtained.

> The timing of puberty is influenced by nutritional, genetic, ethnic and environmental factors.

Physical examination: Detailed anthropometrics, sexual maturity, dysmorphic features suggestive of any syndromes, presence of gynecomastia, micropenis, sense of smell.

Biochemical/Hormonal assessment:
- Plasma testosterone or estradiol
- Plasma follicle-stimulating hormone (FSH) and luteinizing hormone (LH)
- Bone age X-ray
- Tests of olfaction.

Further studies that may be indicated are:
- Magnetic resonance imaging (MRI) with contrast enhancement to rule out any pituitary or hypothalamic pathology
- GnRH or GnRH agonist stimulation test
- Visual acuity and visual fields
- Karyotype
- Pelvic/abdominal ultrasonography.

Other hormonal evaluation (usually in males):
- Assessment of hCG stimulation of testosterone levels
- AMH (anti-Müllerian hormone)
- Inhibin B
- Evaluation of other pituitary axes—plasma thyroxine, thyroid-stimulating hormone (TSH)
- Cortisol, IGF-1, prolactin

Q. 5 Name some causes of each type of hypogonadism.

Ans.

> For boys undergoing radiotherapy or chemotherapy for any cancers, precautions to be taken.
> - Shield testes from irradiation
> - Testicular function evaluation after treatment for cancer
> - Storage of sperm prior to chemotherapy or radiation treatment in postpubertal males
> - Testosterone replacement as indicated.

Hypergonadotropic hypogonadism: Turner's syndrome, gonadal dysgenesis, gonadal dysfunction due to chemotherapy or radiation therapy.

Hypogonadotropic hypogonadism:
- Tumors—prolactinomas, craniopharyngiomas, Rathke's cleft cysts.
- GnRH deficiency (isolated hypogonadotropic hypogonadism, Kallmann's syndrome), multiple pituitary hormone deficiency (MPHD)
- Infiltrative diseases of the central nervous system—hemochromatosis, sarcoidosis, granulomatous diseases, lymphocytic hypophysitis
- *Infections:* Tuberculosis, HIV/AIDS, syphilis
- Cranial irradiation
- *Trauma:* Pituitary stalk transaction, hypophysectomy
- *Vascular:* Ischemia, Sheehan's syndrome, pituitary apoplexy
- *Drugs:* Opioids, anabolic steroids, corticoids, narcotics
- Functional gonadotropin deficiency secondary to systemic illnesses.

Q. 6 Name some syndromes associated with hypogonadism.

Ans.
- Kallmann syndrome
- Congenital hypogonadotropic hypogonadism with adrenal insufficiency (due to DAX1 mutation)
- Multiple pituitary hormone deficiency (MPHD)
- Prader-Willi syndrome
- Laurence-Moon-Biedl
- CHARGE (Coloboma, heart defect, atresia choanae, retarded growth and development, genital hypoplasia, ear anomalies or deafness)
- Gordon Holmes syndrome—congenital hypogonadotropic hypogonadism (CHH) with cerebral ataxia.

Goals of intervention in delayed puberty
- Determine site and etiology of abnormality if any
- Induce and maintain secondary sexual characteristics
- Induce pubertal growth spurt
- Prevent the potential psychological, and social problems due to delayed puberty
- Normal libido
- Maintain fertility where feasible.

Q. 7 What are the options available to treat hypogonadism?

Ans.
- For primary hypogonadism, replacement with gender appropriate sex steroid
- For hypogonadotropic hypogonadism treatment options are:
- Replacement with sex steroids, or
- Gonadotropins (either as a combination of hCG and human menopausal gonadotropins [hMG] or
- Pulsatile GnRH therapy.

Q. 8 Are there ways to differentiate constitutional delay of growth and puberty (CDGP) from hypogonadotropic hypogonadism (HH)?

Ans. Inhibin B >35 pg/mL and anti-Müllerian hormone (AMH) >110 pmol/L are more frequent in CDGP than in hypogonadism in prepubertal boys.

Stimulation tests such as assessment of gonadotropin response to gonadotropin releasing hormone (GnRH) and testosterone response to human chorionic gonadotropin (hCG) have also been utilized.

> Constitutional delay of puberty should be ruled out before a diagnosis and treatment of hypogonadism.

Q. 9 What is the approach to management of constitutional delay of puberty?

Ans. Any patient with pubertal delay should be assessed for any organic causes leading to delay. CDGP is considered a diagnosis of exclusion, and is confirmed if the patient spontaneously progresses through puberty. A family history of delayed puberty may be present in CDGP. Treatment with low dose sex steroids (50–100 mg of testosterone enanthate, cypionate or proprinoate every 4 weeks for about 3-6 months, with a repeat course of treatment if necessary) may be tried. In girls, 2–5 μg ethinyl estradiol or equivalent low doses of 17β-estradiol or transdermal estrogen or conjugated estrogens everyday for about 6 months may be tried to induce pubertal onset.

Q. 10 What are some suggested hormone replacement regimens in girls?

Ans.

- Hormonal replacement therapy is usually begun around 11–12 years of age.
- Ethinyl estradiol 5 μg (or lower) by mouth or conjugated estrogen 0.3 mg (or less) by mouth daily for 4–6 months or transdermal estradiol, 0.1 μg/kg/day patch is usually started, with gradual increase in doses over two years to adult replacement doses of 20 μg/day ethinyl estradiol or 1.25 mg/day conjugated estrogen or 100 μg/day transdermal estradiol.
- After about 2 years of estrogen or when patient develops breakthrough bleeding, progestin is added. Hormones are given cyclically with estrogen for the first 21 days of the month and 200–300 mg micronized oral progesterone or 5 mg oral medroxyprogesterone for about 12 days a month from day 10 to day 21. A 7-day pill free period leads to monthly menstrual bleeding.
- Once patient has attained adult replacement doses and is having regular cycles, she may be switched to oral contraceptive preparations containing combination of estrogen and progesterone.

Q. 11 What are some suggested hormone replacement regimens in boys?

Ans. Long acting testosterone esters (enanthate or cypionate) started at a dose of 25–50 mg injected intramuscularly every 3–4 weeks with 50 mg increments every 6–9 months till an adult maintenance dose (200–250 mg every 3–4 weeks) is reached.

The goals of testosterone treatment involve stimulating physical puberty, virilization, attainment of normal muscle mass and bone mineral density for age, and psychosocial wellbeing.

Q. 12 Are there potentially reversible causes of hypogonadism?

Ans. Transient or functional hypogonadotropic hypogonadism—chronic systemic diseases such as inflammatory bowel disease, celiac disease, anorexia nervosa or bulimia, malnutrition, obesity, diabetes mellitus, Cushing's syndrome, hypothyroidism, hyperprolactinemia, autoimmune disorders, nephrotic syndrome, sickle cell disease, thalassemia, alcoholism, excessive exercise, etc.

Q. 13 What are the forms of testosterone preparations available for therapy?

Ans. Testosterone enanthate or cypionate—IM injections usually administered every 2–4 weeks.

Testosterone undecanoate injections—long-acting injections administered once every 3 months.

Testosterone gel, transdermal testosterone patches, testosterone oral pills, subcutaneously placed testosterone pellets are other forms of treatment.

Q. 14 What forms of estrogen and progesterone are available?

Ans. Transdermal estrogens (TDE), oral estradiol or ethinyl estradiol or conjugated equine estrogens (CEE) are available for therapy. The equivalence of daily doses are 100 μg TDE or 2 mg oral estradiol or 20 μg ethinyl estradiol or 1.25 mg CEE or injectable estradiol cypionate, 2.5 mg/month.

Micronized oral progestogens or medroxyprogesterone are commonly used progesterones. Other progesterones part of combined oral contraceptives are levonorgestrel, desogestrel, etc.

Follow-up of clinical case: Patient undergoes MRI brain noting hypoplasia of anterior pituitary gland and ectopic posterior pituitary bright spot. Patient is diagnosed with panhypopituitarism and initiated on thyroid and growth hormone replacement with plan to induce puberty once he achieves a height close to 3%. Patient is also instructed on stress dose hydrocortisone coverage in case of illness.

SUGGESTED READING

1. Bhasin S, Cunningham GR, Hayes FJ, et al. Testosterone therapy in men with androgen deficiency syndromes: an Endocrine Society clinical practice guideline. J Clin Endocrinol Metabol. 2010;95:2536-59.
2. Bondy CA. Care of girls and women with Turner syndrome: a guideline of the Turner Syndrome Study Group. J Clin Endocrinol Metabol. 2007;92:10-25.
3. Davenport ML. Approach to the patient with Turner syndrome. J Clin Endocrinol Metabol. 2010;95:1487-95.
4. Dunkel L, Quinton R. Transition in endocrinology: induction of puberty. European Journal of Endocrinology/European Federation of Endocrine Societies. 2014;170: R229-39.
5. Harrington J, Palmert MR. Clinical review: Distinguishing constitutional delay of growth and puberty from isolated hypogonadotropic hypogonadism: critical appraisal of available diagnostic tests. J Clin Endocrinol Metabol. 2012;97:3056-67.

6. Palmert MR, Dunkel L. Clinical practice. Delayed puberty. New England J Med. 2012;366:443-53.
7. Raivio T, Falardeau J, Dwyer A, et al. Reversal of idiopathic hypogonadotropic hypogonadism. New England J Med. 2007;357:863-73.
8. Silveira LF, Latronico AC. Approach to the patient with hypogonadotropic hypogonadism. J Clin Endocrinol Metabol. 2013;98:1781-8.
9. Villanueva C, Argente J. Pathology or normal variant: what constitutes a delay in puberty? Hormone Research in Paediatrics. 2014;82:213-21.
10. Young J. Approach to the male patient with congenital hypogonadotropic hypogonadism. J Clin Endocrinol Metabol. 2012;97:707-18.

CHAPTER

6

Approach to Subclinical Hypothyroidism

Pramila Kalra

CASE

A 26-year-old female presents with the complaints of weight gain of 5 kg in the past 5 months. She also has complaints of arthralgias, lethargy and fatigue. Her body mass index (BMI) is 30 kg/m^2.

She has one child and is not planning for conception in the near future.

She is advised thyroid stimulating hormone (TSH) test which shows a value of 7 mIU/L. Her T4 is 6.5 ug/dL and she has come for the treatment of hypothyroidism. She thinks that her weight gain is solely due to hypothyroidism.

On detailed history, her daily calories intake is averaged about 2200 kcal/day and is predominantly rich in carbohydrates. Her fiber intake in the diet is very poor. She is a pure vegetarian.

She is hardly going out in the sunlight and uses sunscreen with a sun protection factor of 40 when she goes out in the sunlight. Her average calcium intake in the diet with a 7-day recall history is about 400 mg per day.

On examination, she has no typical features suggestive of hypothyroidism except for rubbery consistency of the goiter, which is smooth and 1.5 times enlarged.

What is the treatment approach for this patient?

Q. 1 What should be done in this patient?

Ans. Patients with primary hypothyroidism with TSH levels above 10 mIU/L should be treated but whether patients with TSH levels of 4.5–10 mIU/L will benefit from therapy is less certain.

Q. 2 What are the possible benefits of treating subclinical hypothyroidism?

Ans. Some studies have shown a beneficial response in atherosclerosis risk factors such as atherogenic lipids, impaired endothelial and intima media thickness. The epicardial adipose tissue has been shown to be increased in patients with subclinical hypothyroidism and this could be associated with possible cardiovascular adverse effects of subclinical hypothyroidism.

Q. 3 What is the relationship of hypothyroidism to weight gain?

Ans. The appetite in those with marked hypothyroidism is often suppressed which offsets the impact of a decrease in metabolic rate and so myxedema may present with weight loss, and overt hypothyroidism does not appear to be more common in the obese population than in the general population. Subclinical hypothyroidism can cause approximately 0.8 kg of weight gain. The weight loss which happens post-treatment in patients with hypothyroidism is due to fluid mobilization.

Q. 4 What is the relationship of hypothyroidism to obesity?

Ans. Obesity may cause a relatively elevated TSH because of the probable impact on the hypothalamic-pituitary-thyroid axis. These patients may have ultrasound findings suggestive of chronic thyroiditis without either elevated antithyroid antibody titers or decreased T4 and T3 levels. So we should be cautious when diagnosing subclinical hypothyroidism in the setting of marked obesity.

The above-mentioned lady should be specifically counseled about lifestyle modification and should be told that her weight gain cannot be solely attributed to hypothyroidism.

Q. 5 What is the upper limit of normal range of TSH?

Ans. The reference range of a given laboratory should determine the upper limit of normal for a third generation TSH assay. The normal TSH reference range changes with age. If an age-based upper limit of normal for a third generation TSH assay is not available in an iodine sufficient area, an upper limit of normal of 4.12 should be considered.

Q. 6 What are the indications of treatment of subclinical hypothyroidism?

Ans. If patients have symptoms suggestive of hypothyroidism, positive thyroid peroxidase antibody (TPOAb) or evidence of atherosclerotic cardiovascular disease, heart failure, or associated risk factors for these diseases. If a women who is pregnant or planning for conception in near future pregnancy specific cut-offs should be used for deciding about starting treatment (Boxes 6.1 and 6.2).

The above patient is subjected to testing of TPOAb and the levels are found to be >1300 U/L.

The patient is diagnosed as Hashimotos thyroiditis and hence is started on levothyroxine supplementation in view of the TPOAb positivity and presence of goiter in a dose of 25 μg daily in the morning.

She is advised lifestyle modification and counseled about it and told that her weight gain cannot be attributed to hypothyroidism alone.

BOX 6.1 Other autoimmune disorders associated with Hashimoto's thyroiditis

- Type 1 diabetes
- Pernicious anemia
- Primary adrenal failure (Addison's disease)
- Myasthenia gravis
- Celiac disease
- Rheumatoid arthritis
- Systemic lupus erythematosis and rarely thyroid lymphoma

BOX 6.2 Reference ranges for TSH in pregnancy	
• First trimester	Up to 4 mIU/L if TPO negative and 2.5 mIU/L if TPO positive and high risk pregnancy
• Second trimester	Up to 4 mIU/L if TPO negative and 3 mIU/L if TPO positive OR high risk pregnancy
• Third trimester	Up to 4 mIU/L if TPO negative and 3 mIU/L if TPO positive OR high risk pregnancy

Q. 7 When is the TSH value lowest and highest?

Ans. The TSH values tend to be lowest in the late afternoon and highest around the hour of sleep (Box 6.3).

Is very mild elevation of TSH value in very old age always a reflection of subclinical hypothyroidism?

Very mild elevations of TSH in older individuals may not reflect subclinical hypothyroidism but it may be a part of normal aging.

Q. 8 When should antithyroid peroxidase antibodies be measured?

Ans. Antithyroid peroxidase antibodies should be measured when evaluating patients with subclinical hypothyroidism, to diagnose autoimmune thyroiditis when nodular goiter is present and during evaluation of patients with recurrent miscarriages whether or not they have infertility.

Q. 9 What is the role of TSH receptor antibodies (TSHRAbs) measurement in patients with hypothyroidism?

Ans. The TSH receptor antibodies (TSHRAbs) using a sensitive assay should be considered in hypothyroid pregnant patients with a history of Graves' disease who were treated with radioactive iodine or thyroidectomy prior to pregnancy. This should be initially done either at 20–26 weeks of gestation or during the first trimester.

Q. 10 What should be used for the treatment of hypothyroidism?

Ans. Levothyroxine is the recommended treatment of choice for treatment of hypothyroidism.

Q. 11 What is the dose recommendation for subclinical hypothyroidism?

Ans. Patients with subclinical hypothyroidism will require a dose of 25–75 μg daily which is usually sufficient for achieving euthyroid levels and larger doses are usually required for those presenting with higher TSH values.

Q. 12 How much gap is needed for proper absorption of the tablet?

Ans. The best absorption happens if taken 60 minutes prior to the breakfast or 4 hours after the last meal but because of compliance patients are told to keep a gap between 30 and 60 minutes before breakfast after taking the tablet with water (Box 6.4).

Q. 13 When should the patients be retested?

Ans. The repeat testing for TSH should be done after 8 weeks of starting the therapy.

BOX 6.3 TSH secretion affected by effect on hypothalamic pituitary axis

Decrease
- Bexarotene
- Dopamine
- Dopaminergic agonists (bromocriptine, cabergoline)
- Glucocorticoids
- Thyroid hormone analogs somatostatin analogs (octreotide, lanreotide)
- Metformin
- Opiates (e.g. heroin)
- Interleukin-6

Increase
- Dopamine receptor blockers (metoclopramide)
- Hypoadrenalism
- Interleukin 2
- Amphetamine
- Ritonavir
- St. John's worts

BOX 6.4 Agents that interfere with absorption of levothyroxine

- Bile acid sequestrants (cholestyramine, colestipol, colesevelam)
- Sucralfate cation-exchange resins (Kayexalate)
- Oral bisphosphonates
- Proton pump inhibitors
- Raloxifene
- Multivitamins (containing ferrous sulfate or calcium carbonate)
- Ferrous sulphate
- Phosphate binders (sevelamer, aluminum hydroxide)
- Calcium salts (carbonate, citrate, acetate) chromium picolinate
- Charcoal
- Orlistat
- Ciprofloxacin
- H_2 receptor antagonist
- Malabsorption syndromes
- Celiac disease
- Jejunoileal bypass surgery
- Cirrhosis (biliary)
- Achlorhydria diet
- Ingestion with a meal
- Grapefruit juice
- Expresso coffee
- High fiber diet
- Soyabean formula (infants)
- Soy products

Q. 14 What is the normal range for TSH value recommended in a nonpregnant adult?

Ans. The normal range for TSH value is 4.12 mIU/L based on NHANES III data.

Q. 15 Do elderly patients require more or less levothyroxine supplementation?

Ans. The elderly patients absorb L-thyroxine less efficiently and they often require 20–25% less per kilogram daily than younger patients, due to decreased lean body mass.

Q. 16 If free T4 has to be checked for monitoring of hypothyroidism when should it be collected?

Ans. In monitoring patients with hypothyroidism on L-thyroxine replacement, blood for assessment of serum free T4 should be collected before dosing because the level will be transiently increased by up to 20% after L-thyroxine administration in a study of athyreotic patients it was seen that serum total T4 levels increased above baseline by 1 hour and peaked at 2.5 hours, while serum free T4 levels peaked at 3.5 hours and remained higher than baseline for 9 hours.

Q. 17 Which is a better monitoring tool in pregnancy T4 or FT4?

Ans. In pregnancy, measurement of serum total T4 is recommended over direct immunoassay of serum free T4 as due to alterations in serum proteins in pregnancy, direct immunoassay of free T4 may yield lower values based on reference ranges established with normal nonpregnant sera.

Q. 18 Do we need to any further tests at this point of time for her?

Ans. She has a history of poor exposure to sunlight and hence she is tested for vitamin D deficiency and her vitamin D levels are found to be 4 ng/mL.

She is started on vitamin D supplementation and also on calcium supplementation in view of her poor calcium intake in the diet.

In view of her being a pure vegetarian her vitamin B_{12} levels are also checked which are found to be 140 ng/L and she is also started on vitamin B_{12} supplements.

Q. 19 Is there any association of vitamin D deficiency with subclinical hypothyroidism?

Ans. The coexistence of subclinical hypothyroidism with vitamin D deficiency can lead to further deterioration in the LV diastolic function via the regulation of intracellular calcium and induction of inflammatory activity.

Q. 20 What is the role of L-tyrosine?

Ans. L-tyrosine has been touted as a treatment for hypothyroidism by virtue of its role in thyroid hormone synthesis. There are no preclinical or clinical studies demonstrating that L-tyrosine has thyromimetic properties. B vitamins, garlic, ginger, gingko, licorice, magnesium, manganese, meadowsweet, oats, pineapple, potassium, saw palmetto, and valerian are included in various commercially available "thyroid-enhancing preparations". But studies have not shown any beneficial effect.

Q. 21 What is the role of selenium?

Ans. There is presently not enough data to support the use of selenium for treatment or prevention of hypothyroidism.

Q. 22 What is the recommended frequency of screening in adults who are euthyroid?

Ans. The American thyroid association recommends screening of all men and women who are above 35 years of age every 5 years.

Follow-up of the Case

The lady comes back for follow-up after 2 months. She has lost 3.8 kg of weight and has started rigorous lifestyle modification. Her repeat TSH is 3.5 mIU/L and she is asked to come for follow-up after six months and continue with the same treatment.

SUGGESTED READING

1. Alexander EK, Pearce EN, Brent GA, Brown RS, Chen H, Dosiou C, et al. 2017 Guidelines of the American Thyroid Association for the Diagnosis and Management of Thyroid Disease During Pregnancy and the Postpartum. Thyroid. 2017;27(3): 315-389.
2. Andersen MN, Olsen AM, Madsen JC, Faber J, Torp-Pedersen C, Gislason GH, et al. Levothyroxine substitution in patients with subclinical hypothyroidism and the risk of myocardial infarction and mortality. PLoS One. 2015;10(6).
3. Belen E, Değirmencioğlu A, Zencirci E, Tipi FF, Altun Ö, Karakuş G, et al. The association between subclinical hypothyroidism and epicardial adipose tissue thickness. Korean Circ J. 2015;45(3):210-5.
4. Duntas LH, Brabant G, Monzani F, Pearce SH, Peeters RP, Razvi S, et al. Reply on the Letter by Stott, et al. 'The Dilemma of Treating Subclinical Hypothyroidism: Risk that Current Guidelines Do More Harm than Good.' Eur Thyroid J. 2014;3(2):139-40. doi: 10.1159/000360622. Epub. 2014.
5. Garber JR, Cobin RH, Gharib H, Hennessey JV, Klein I, Mechanick JI, et al. American Association of Clinical Endocrinologists and American Thyroid Association Taskforce on Hypothyroidism in Adults. Clinical practice guidelines for hypothyroidism in adults: cosponsored by the American Association of Clinical Endocrinologists and the American Thyroid Association. Endocr Pract. 2012;18(6):988-1028. Erratum in: Endocr Pract. 2013;19(1):175.
6. Lazarus J, Brown RS, Daumerie C, Hubalewska-Dydejczyk A, Negro R, Vaidya B. 2014 European thyroid association guidelines for the management of subclinical hypothyroidism in pregnancy and in children. Eur Thyroid J. 2014;3(2):76-94.
7. Mooradian AD. Subclinical hypothyroidism in the elderly: to treat or not to treat? Am J Ther. 2011;18(6):477-86. doi: 10.1097/MJT.0b013e3181e0ca9c.
8. Review Chan S, Boelaert K. Optimal management of hypothyroidism, hypothyroxinaemia and euthyroid TPO antibody positivity preconception and in pregnancy. Clin Endocrinol (Oxf). 2015;82(3):313-26. doi: 10.1111/cen.12605. Epub. 2014.
9. Rosario PW, Calsolari MR. How selective are the new guidelines for treatment of subclinical hypothyroidism for patients with thyrotropin levels at or below 10 mIU/L? Thyroid. 2013;23(5):562-5.
10. Yilmaz H, Cakmak M, Darcin T, Inan O, Gurel OM, Bilgic MA, et al. Subclinical hypothyroidism in combination with vitamin D deficiency increases the risk of impaired left ventricular diastolic function. Endocr Regul. 2015;49(2):84-90.

CHAPTER

7

Approach to Thyrotoxicosis

Chitra S

CASE 1

A 30-year-old woman presents with complaints of palpitations, tremulousness and weight loss of around 4 kg (despite a good appetite) over the last 2 months. On examination, she is anxious, has a pulse rate of 100/min, warm and moist peripheries, fine tremors of the outstretched hands and a visible goiter. No obvious abnormalities in the eyes. Her last menstrual period was 15 days ago. Her primary care physician orders for laboratory examination which reveals normal hemogram with an erythrocyte sedimentation rate of 25 mm in the first hour. Thyroid stimulating hormone (TSH) <0.001 μIU/L and total T4 28 μg/dL.

A diagnosis of thyrotoxicosis is made. She is started on beta-blockers and she is asked to get a technetium uptake scan and review.

Q. 1 What is the typical thyroid profile seen in a patient with thyrotoxicosis?

Ans. The relationship between free T4 and TSH (when the pituitary-thyroid axis is intact) is an inverse log-linear relationship; therefore, small changes in free T4 result in large changes in serum TSH concentrations. Thus, suppressed TSH levels are considerably more sensitive than direct thyroid hormone measurements for assessing thyroid hormone excess states.

A suppressed TSH level with normal or elevated T4 and/or T3 levels are characteristic of thyroid hormone excess (exogenous or endogenous).

- Thyrotoxicosis refers to the clinical syndrome of hypermetabolism due to excessive circulating thyroid hormones.
- Hyperthyroidism is the sustained increase in thyroid hormone biosynthesis.

Q. 2 Of the various causes, which are the most common causes of thyrotoxicosis?

Ans. The most common cause of thyrotoxicosis is Graves' disease accounting for close to 60–90%. The remaining cases are caused by toxic adenoma or multinodular goiter and thyroiditis.

Q. 3 How can one differentiate clinically between subacute thyroiditis, Graves' disease and toxic multinodular goiters?

Ans. Certain features give clues to the underlying etiology of thyrotoxicosis

- Duration of symptoms
- Size, shape of thyroid gland
- Presence or absence of tenderness over thyroid
- Extrathyroidal manifestations of Graves' disease.

Graves' disease usually occurs in patients with a family history, has been symptomatic for several weeks to months, have a diffuse goiter, and has symptoms related to extrathyroidal manifestations of Graves', most commonly ophthalmopathy like feeling of grittiness in the eyes, increasing prominence of eyes. In severe instances, a thyroid bruit can be appreciated over the thyroid.

Patients with toxic multinodular goiter are generally older, have had the swelling in front of the neck for many years, have been symptomatic for months and have a nodular goiter with no extrathyroidal features like in Graves'.

Subacute thyroiditis mostly have symptoms lasting from few days to weeks, is generally painful, the gland is firm to hard on palpation, and the erythrocyte sedimentation rate (ESR) is almost always >50 and sometimes over 100 mm/h.

That being said, it helps to be mindful that not all patients with Graves' have extrathyroidal features, and about 10% of them might not have a palpable goiter. Not all nodular goiters are toxic multinodular goiters. These are just pointers to suggest one cause more than the other.

Q. 4 When do we ask for a radioiodine scan/technetium scan in a patient with thyrotoxicosis?

Ans. An uptake study should be asked for when clinical presentation is not diagnostic of Graves' disease. An uptake scan is added when thyroid nodularity is noted.

Q. 5 What is the principle of the uptake study?

Ans. A radioactive iodine uptake (RAIU) is indicated when the diagnosis is in question. If the thyroid gland is hyperactive, then the uptake of radioiodine is elevated (like in Graves' and toxic multinodular goiter). Whereas in conditions like thyroiditis, the uptake is close to zero.

Amongst conditions with increased uptake, the pattern of uptake (in a scan study) will help differentiate. The pattern of RAIU in GD is diffuse, unless there are coexistent nodules or fibrosis.

The pattern of uptake in a patient with a single TA generally shows focal uptake in the adenoma with suppressed uptake in the surrounding and contralateral thyroid tissue. The image in TMNG demonstrates multiple areas of focal increased and suppressed uptake.

Q. 6 What is Technetium 99 scan? Is it the same as radioiodine?

Ans. Both are molecules that are rapidly taken up by the sodium iodine symporter (NIS) in the thyroid gland. Technetium offers the advantage of imaging in 20 min, lesser radiation exposure and easier accessibility as compared to ^{123}I. Thus, in the differential diagnosis of thyrotoxicosis, more centers are using technetium than radioiodine.

Q. 7 What is an absolute contraindication for a radioiodine scan?

Ans. Pregnancy is an absolute contraindication for a radioiodine scan.

Q. 8 Why is it relevant to know whether the thyrotoxicosis is due to thyroiditis or other causes?

Ans. Thyroiditis is a condition where stored thyroid hormones are released secondary to destruction of the thyroid gland and is usually for a period of 1–3 months. The symptoms are managed with beta blockers alone. There is no role of antithyroid drugs in thyroiditis as there is no hyperfunctioning of the gland. Hence, the need to make the distinction as it affects treatment modality and prognosis.

Q. 9 Why is the role of beta blockers in the management of thyrotoxicosis?

Ans. Beta-adrenergic blockade should be considered in all patients with symptomatic thyrotoxicosis.

Treatment with beta blockers leads to a decrease in heart rate, systolic blood pressure, muscle weakness, and tremor, as well as improvement in the degree of irritability, emotional lability, and exercise intolerance. Propranolol is a nonselective beta blocker most used in thyrotoxicosis, usually in the doses of 10–40 mg qid to tid. At high doses, it may reduce T4 to T3 conversion. Other beta blockers used are atenolol and metoprolol. Caution should be exercised in patients with bronchospasm before starting beta blockers. Calcium-channel blockers, verapamil and diltiazem can be used in patients in whom beta blockers are contraindicated.

Q. 10 When do we start antithyroid drugs for a patient with thyrotoxicosis?

Ans. Antithyroid drugs are used in patients of thyrotoxicosis secondary to hyperthyroidism. This class of drugs reduce the production of thyroid hormones by inhibiting iodine oxidation and organification of tyrosine residues in thyroglobulin.

In India, methimazole, its precursor carbimazole and propylthiouracil are available. 10 mg of carbimazole is equivalent to 6 mg of methimazole. Carbimazole/methimazole is the preferred agent while propylthiouracil is reserved for special situations like first trimester of pregnancy or thyroid storm.

Q. 11 How are antithyroid drugs initiated in a patient with hyperthyroidism?

Ans. It is prudent to get a baseline complete blood count, including white count with differential, and a liver profile including bilirubin and transaminases. A baseline absolute neutrophil count $<500/mm^3$ or liver transaminases enzyme levels elevated more than five-fold the upper limit of normal are contraindications to initiating antithyroid drug therapy. Carbimazole and methimazole are started at a dose of 10–20 mg/day and has the advantage of being administered once daily. Propylthiouracil (PTU) has a shorter duration of action and is usually administered two or three times daily, starting with 50–150 mg three times daily.

The 2016 American Thyroid Association guidelines suggests the following as a rough guide to initial MMI daily dosing: 5–10 mg if free T4 is 1–1.5 times the upper limit of normal; 10–20 mg for free T4 1.5–2 times the upper limit of normal;

and 30–40 mg for free T4 2–3 times the upper limit of normal. These rough guidelines should be tailored to the individual patient, incorporating additional information on symptoms, gland size, and total T3 levels where relevant.

Q. 12 What are the common side effects of antithyroid drugs?

Ans. The minor side effects include urticaria, arthralgia, arthritis, fever, transient granulocytopenia, gastrointestinal upset and alterations in taste and smell.

The major side effects include agranulocytosis, and very rarely aplastic anemia, thrombocytopenia, toxic hepatitis (PTU), cholestatic hepatitis (MMI), vasculitis, hypoprothrombinemia (PTU), hypoglycemia due to anti-insulin antibodies (MMI) and pancreatitis (MMI).

Q. 13 What are the instructions to be given to a patient on antithyroid drugs?

Ans. Patients need to educated at initiation and at every subsequent visit to stop the drug immediately and report back, if they notice pruritic rash, jaundice, acholic stools or dark urine, arthralgias, abdominal pain, nausea, fatigue, fever, or pharyngitis (suggestive of agranulocytosis or hepatic injury).

Q. 14 How do you monitor a patient on antithyroid drugs?

Ans. An assessment of serum free T4 and total T3 should be obtained about 2–6 weeks after initiation of therapy, depending on the severity of the thyrotoxicosis, and the dose of medication should be adjusted accordingly. The dose of antithyroid drugs adjusted accordingly. Once the patient is euthyroid, the dose of MMI can usually be decreased by 30–50%, and biochemical testing repeated in 4–6 weeks. TSH can remain suppressed even after normalization of T4 and T3 levels, hence is not the ideal parameter for monitoring.

Q. 15 How do we monitor for adverse effects of antithyroid drugs?

Ans. Most patients who develop agranulocytosis are symptomatic, hence a differential white blood cell count should be obtained during febrile illness and at the onset of pharyngitis in all patients taking antithyroid medication.

Similarly, liver function should be assessed in patients who experience pruritic rash, jaundice, light-colored stool or dark urine, joint pain, abdominal pain or bloating, anorexia, nausea, or fatigue.

There is insufficient evidence to recommend for or against routine monitoring of WBC counts and liver function tests in patients taking ATDs.

Q. 16 How do you manage a patient who has developed adverse effects of ATD?

Ans. Minor cutaneous reactions may be managed with concurrent antihistamine therapy without stopping the antithyroid drug (ATD). Any patient who develops agranulocytosis or other serious side effects while taking either MMI or PTU, use of the other medication is generally contraindicated owing to risk of cross-reactivity between the two medications.

Q. 17 How long does a patient need to stay on antithyroid drugs?

Ans. Once the patient is rendered euthyroid, the dose of antithyroid drug is tapered and continued for 12–18 months and discontinued if TSH is normal. The reasoning behind the recommendation is that the remission rates are not higher even, if ATD are continued for longer than 18 months. The patient is said to be in remission, if the TSH, TT4 and TT3 are normal one year after discontinuation of ATD. Patients with small goiters, mild disease and negative TSH receptor antibody (TRAb) are more likely to have remission. Males, smokers, patients with large goiters and persistently high TSH receptor antibody have higher relapse rates. Continued low-dose MMI treatment for longer than 12–18 months may be considered in patients not in remission who prefer this approach.

Q. 18 How do you follow-up a patient in whom ATD drugs were stopped?

Ans. Thyroid function should be assessed at 1–3 months for 6–12 months after stopping ATD to diagnose relapse promptly. Patients should also be informed to report back, if symptoms of hyperthyroidism develop.

Q. 19 What are the options available as definitive treatment for Graves' disease?

Ans. Once patient is rendered euthyroid, definitive therapy in the form of surgery (thyroidectomy) or radioiodine ablation can be offered to the patient. The modality of treatment is selected is based on patient characteristics and preferences. Low dose antithyroid drugs can also be continued long-term in some patients.

Q. 20 When is surgery preferred as a definitive treatment?

Ans. Patients who have compressive symptoms such as dysphagia, difficulty breathing or change in voice, or patients with large goiters, have a nodule suspicious of malignancy, patients who have moderate-to-severe active Graves' orbitopathy, (where radioiodine can worsen condition), or patients planning pregnancy within 4–6 months are candidates ideal for surgery.

Patients with substantial coexisting comorbidities make poor candidates for surgery.

Q. 21 Who are ideal candidate for radioiodine ablation?

Ans. Patients with substantial comorbidities making them poor candidates for surgery, patients with past history of neck surgery or irradiation (making surgery difficult), patients who develop adverse effects to ATD are suitable candidates for radioablation.

Pregnancy, breastfeeding, moderate-severe active Graves' orbitopathy, co-existing thyroid cancer or suspicion of the same and patients who cannot comply with postablation safety regulations are contraindications for radioablation.

Q. 22 Should all patients receive ATD prior to administration of radioiodine?

Ans. Because RAI treatment of GD can cause a transient exacerbation of hyperthyroidism, beta-adrenergic blockade should be considered even in asymptomatic patients who are at increased risk for complications due to worsening of hyperthyroidism (i.e. elderly patients and patients with comorbidities.

Patients who are extremely symptomatic, elderly and with comorbidities that can worsen with increasing thyroid hormone levels and have free T4 levels 2–3 times upper limit of normal are usually candidates for pretreatment with methimazole. ATD should be stopped at least 3–5 days prior to radioiodine administration.

Q. 23 How is the dose of radioiodine ^{131}I calculated?

Ans. The goal of treatment is to render the patient hypothyroid. The dose can be calculated using the formula. This formula needs determination of uptake at 24 hrs and the estimation of the weight of the thyroid gland by the physician.

$$\text{Dose of } ^{131}\text{I} = \frac{50\text{–}120\ \mu\text{Ci} \times \text{weight of thyroid in grams}}{24 \text{ hour uptake}}$$

The other method involves administration of a fixed dose ranging from 10 to 15 mCi.

Q. 24 What are the precautions to be taken prior to radioiodine ablation?

Ans. A urine pregnancy test should be done 48 hours prior to radioablation in any female with child-bearing potential. Detailed written instructions should be handed to the patient.

Q. 25 What are the adverse effects of radioiodine ablation?

Ans. Patients are to be educated that hypothyroidism postablation is to be expected. Radiation thyroiditis presenting with anterior neck pain occurs rarely and is usually mild. Concerns about thyroid malignancy and other tumors, reduced fertility postablation, increased cardiovascular and cancer mortality exist, although no conclusive evidence for the same exist.

Q. 26 How does one follow-up a patient after radioablation?

Ans. Patient is called for review after 1–2 months with free T4 and total T3 levels. Most patients are rendered hypothyroid by 4–6 months. The dose of levothyroxine is decided by the free T4 levels. It is important to remember that rarely patient may have transient hypothyroidism following radioactive iodine therapy, with subsequent complete recovery of thyroid function or recurrent hyperthyroidism.

Q. 27 If surgery is the chosen modality of treatment, then what surgery is advisable?

Ans. If surgery is chosen as the therapy, near-total or total thyroidectomy is the procedure of choice.

Q. 28 What are the complications to be anticipated postsurgery?

Ans. The most common complications following near-total or total thyroidectomy are hypocalcemia (which can be transient or permanent), recurrent or superior laryngeal nerve injury (which can be temporary or permanent), postoperative bleeding, and complications related to general anesthesia.

CASE 1 (CONTD...)

Technetium scan reveals diffuse uptake in both lobes of thyroid suggestive of Graves' disease. She is started on antithyroid drugs. She is rendered euthyroid by 6 months and was on 2.5 mg of carbimazole per day. She is planning a pregnancy in the next few months. What is the plan of care for this patient?

As this patient is planning pregnancy in the next few months, she could be offered surgery or continued on ATD. Patient chooses surgery. She had a near total thyroidectomy and was started on levothyroxine 88 μg/day.

CASE 2

A recent educational program conducted in the neighborhood about thyroid disorders and pregnancy has had many pregnant women ask for their thyroid profile as soon as they discover they are pregnant. They come in with their reports for interpretation.

Case 2a

Primigravida with 2.5 months amenorrhea. No family history of thyroid illness. She is feeling well except that she is tired in the evenings. No palpitations, vomiting, weight loss. On examination, pulse is 98/min, no other features of thyrotoxicosis. No goiter.

Urine pregnancy test positive. TSH 0.01 μIU/mL. Total T4 14 μg/dL.

Q. 1 How do we interpret these reports?

Ans. Many physiological changes occur in pregnancy which can cause changes to the parameters, which we normally use to assess thyroid status. Serum TSH levels may be below the nonpregnant reference range in the first half of a normal-term pregnancy, presumably the result of stimulation of the normal thyroid by high levels of serum hCG. Serum total T4 and total T3 levels increase in pregnancy due to the effect of increased estrogen on the thyroid binding globulin. Hence, in pregnancy, the normal limit for total T4 and T3 values are 1.5 times the non-pregnant range.

So this patient's reports appear normal and the changes represent the physiological changes of pregnancy, a free T4 is ordered which was in the normal limit. Hence, she is followed up and her repeat TSH at 5 months is 1.2 μIU/mL.

Case 2b

Here is a patient who is a primigravida with 10 weeks twin gestation. She has nausea and vomiting. She has complaints of tiredness, palpitations and has lost 2 kg since the pregnancy.

On examination, she has a pulse rate of 110/min looks anxious and has fine tremors of extremities. She has a small goiter. Eyes appear normal.

Serum beta hCG >2500 m IU/mL TSH < 0.001 μIU/mL Total T4 30 μg/dL free T4 28 ng/dL.

This patient has hyperthyroidism. The two important causes of hyperthyroidism in early pregnancy are gestational hyperthyroidism and Graves' disease.

Gestational hyperthyroidism is a generally asymptomatic, mild biochemical hyperthyroidism that may be observed in the first trimester of normal pregnancy. It is presumably caused by the high serum hCG of early pregnancy and is not associated with adverse pregnancy outcomes. It is usually self-limited and resolves by 14–16 weeks of gestation. This condition does not warrant the use of antithyroid drugs.

Our patient receives symptomatic treatment in the form of hydration and anti-emetic medication and she improves and her thyroid profile normalizes by the 14th week.

Case 2c

A primigravida with 12 weeks gestation presents with weight loss and palpitations and inability to sleep, she has lost 2 kg since the pregnancy. She has a family history of thyroid illness. She has noticed increased grittiness in both her eyes since the last 6 months. On examination, she has a pulse rate of 120/min, a visible goiter and fine tremors. She has upper eyelid retraction and no obvious proptosis or other eye signs.

Serum β-hCG 450 m IU/mL TSH < 0.001 μ IU/mL, Total T4 225 μg/dL free T4 25 ng/dL.

With the family history of thyroid disease and the eye symptoms, the probability of Graves' disease as the etiology is very high. Uptake scans are contraindicated in pregnancy. Hence, TSH receptor antibody is ordered which is positive. A diagnosis of Graves' disease is made.

Propylthiouracil is the preferred antithyroid agent in the first trimester due to concerns about teratogenic effects of carbimazole. She is started on PTU 50 mg tid and monitored to maintain free T 4 in the upper limit of normal. In the second trimester, she is switched to carbimazole as PTU has reports of fatal hepatic necrosis, and hence is used only for the short period of first trimester when the risk of teratogenic effects of carbimazole are highest.

CASE 3

A 55-year-old male develops complaints of sudden onset persistent diplopia while looking ahead since a week. On questioning, he lets us know that he has had similar complaints of diplopia intermittently, especially on waking up for the last two months which did not interfere with his daily activities. He has also noticed complaints of redness in the right eye and a feeling of grittiness in both eyes. His wife adds that it seems like his eyes are 'popping out' of his sockets.

He has noticed weight loss of around 8% over the last few months with insomnia and fatigue, both of which he attributed to his current change of his boss at work and hence was not investigated for.

His sister has primary hypothyroidism and is on levothyroxine supplements. He is a smoker (20 pack years).

On examination, he is well built, with a BMI of 26 kg/m^2. He appeared anxious, has a pulse rate of 100 bpm, blood pressure of 150/90 mm Hg, warm moist palms, has fine tremors of extremities and a diffuse goiter with no bruit. Eye examination reveals proptosis both eyes (R > L). Lateral movement of the right eye is restricted to 30° from midposition. Clinical activity score was right eye 4/7 (conjunctival redness, pain on movement, chemosis and swelling of the eyelids and the left eye 3/7 (pain on movement,conjunctival redness and chemosis). No dermopathy or nail changes noticed.

TABLE 7.1 Grading of severity of Graves' ophthalmopathy

Grade	*Lid retraction*	*Soft tissues*	*Proptosis*	*Diplopia*	*Corneal exposure*	*Optic nerve status*
Mild	<2 mm	Mild involvement	<3 mm	Transient or absent	Absent	Normal
Moderate	≥2 mm	Moderate involvement	≥3 mm	Inconstant	Mild	Normal
Severe	≥2 mm	Severe involvement	Treatment ≥3 mm	Constant	Mild	Normal
Sight threatening	—	—	—	—	Severe	Compression

Investigations revealed a normal hemogram with normal total and differential leukocyte count. TSH <0.001 μIU/mL, free T4 80 ng/dL. Technetium uptake scan shows diffuse increased uptake over the entire gland.

A diagnosis of Graves' disease with moderate-to-severe, clinically active ophthalmopathy is made.

Q. 1 How is severity of Graves' ophthalmopathy assessed?

Ans. Severity of the Graves' ophthalmopathy is assessed using these parameters like optic nerve status (visual acuity), corneal exposure, diplopia, proptosis, soft tissue involvement and lid retraction as detailed in the Table 7.1.

The severity is graded as sight threatening, moderate-severe and mild. Sight threatening grade involves severe corneal involvement and decrease in visual acuity involving optic nerve compression and is an emergency requiring immediate intervention like intravenous steroids for a short duration and if no improvement is documented, surgical decompression of the orbit.

Moderate-to-severe ophthalmopathy is where is no corneal or optic nerve involvement but proptosis, diplopia, soft tissue involvement and lid retraction are present which may interfere with activities of daily living of the patient.

Mild ophthalmopathy is when the ophthalmopathy has only a minor impact on the life of the patient.

Q. 2 What is clinical activity score?

Ans. It is a seven point score used at the first visit to assess the clinical activity of the ophthalmopathy with each eye receiving one point for the following features:

1. Painful feeling behind the globe over last 4 weeks
2. Pain with eye movement during last 4 weeks
3. Redness of the eyelids
4. Redness of the conjunctiva
5. Swelling of the eyelids
6. Chemosis (edema of the conjunctiva)
7. Swollen caruncle (fleshy body at medial angle of eye).

A score of more than or equal to three indicates clinically active disease in that eye.

Q. 3 Why is it important to assess severity and clinical activity score in ophthalmopathy?

Ans. The severity grading allows the clinician to make decisions about treatment modalities. Sight-threatening ophthalmopathy warrants immediate intervention. Mild ophthalmopathy does not justify the use of immune-based interventions or surgeries. Patients with moderate–severe ophthalmopathy, based on the clinical activity score are categorized in to active and inactive (Flowchart 7.1).

Moderate-severe ophthalmopathy which is active justifies use of steroids while moderate-severe inactive ophthalmopathy needs surgical interventions.

Q. 3a How is sight-threatening ophthalmopathy managed?

Ans. At every follow-up visit, patients need to be asked specifically about a decrease in visual acuity and tested for visual acuity as well. If a drop is noted, urgent referral to an ophthalmologist is to be made to assess visual fields, relative afferent papillary defect and color vision. If dysthyroid optic neuropathy is diagnosed, the patient warrants high dose intravenous glucocorticoids. If no improvements are seen, in a 1–2 weeks time, orbital decompression surgery is to be undertaken.

The second form of sight-threatening ophthalmopathy is corneal breakdown/ ulceration. The role of steroids on corneal breakdown is unknown. Hourly lubrication of the eye, temporary methods to decrease exposure of cornea-like tarsorrhaphy, moisture chamber, or botulinum toxin injection can be tried while orbital decompression is planned at the earliest.

Q. 4 How is active, moderate-to-severe ophthalmopathy managed?

Ans. This group of patients qualify for glucocorticoids to bring down the activity of the disease.

Intravenous glucocorticoids pulses have higher response rates as compared to oral glucocorticoids. Various regimens are used. One of them is 500 mg IV pulses three consecutive days, repeated in 4 monthly cycles with a cumulative dose of 6 g. Higher cumulative doses of IV steroids increase the risk of acute liver injury.

Oral steroids (Prednisolone @ 1 mg/kg/day) also can be initiated for 4–6 weeks and tapered over the next 4 weeks.

Ophthalmopathy may flare up on attempts to withdraw steroids. Screening for conditions that can worsen with steroid therapy is imperative. Bone protection in the form adequate calcium and vitamin D supplementation with or without bisphosphonates are to be provided.

Q. 5 What is the role of orbital radiotherapy in ophthalmopathy?

Ans. In patients with active disease with moderate to severe ophthalmopathy who are not candidates for glucocorticoid therapy or nonresponders to glucocorticoids can be given a trial of radiotherapy. Efficacy of the treatment have been questioned. Diabetes and hypertension are relative contraindications and diabetic retinopathy is an absolute contraindication.

FLOWCHART 7.1 Explaining management of patients with Graves' orbitopathy (GO) based on severity and activity

All patients with GO
• Restore euthyroidism
• Urge smoking withdrawal
• Refer to specialist centers, except for the mildest cases
• Local measures
Mild
Moderate to severe
Sight-threatening (DON)
Local measures wait and see
Progression
Active
Inactive
IV GCs
Poor response (2 weeks)
Stable and inactive
IV GCS (± OR)
Prompt decompression
Still active
Stable and inactive
Rehabilitative surgery (if needed)
Stable and inactive
Rehabilitative surgery
IV GCs (±OR)
Rehabilitative surgery

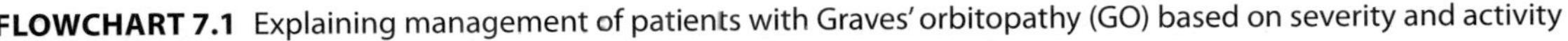

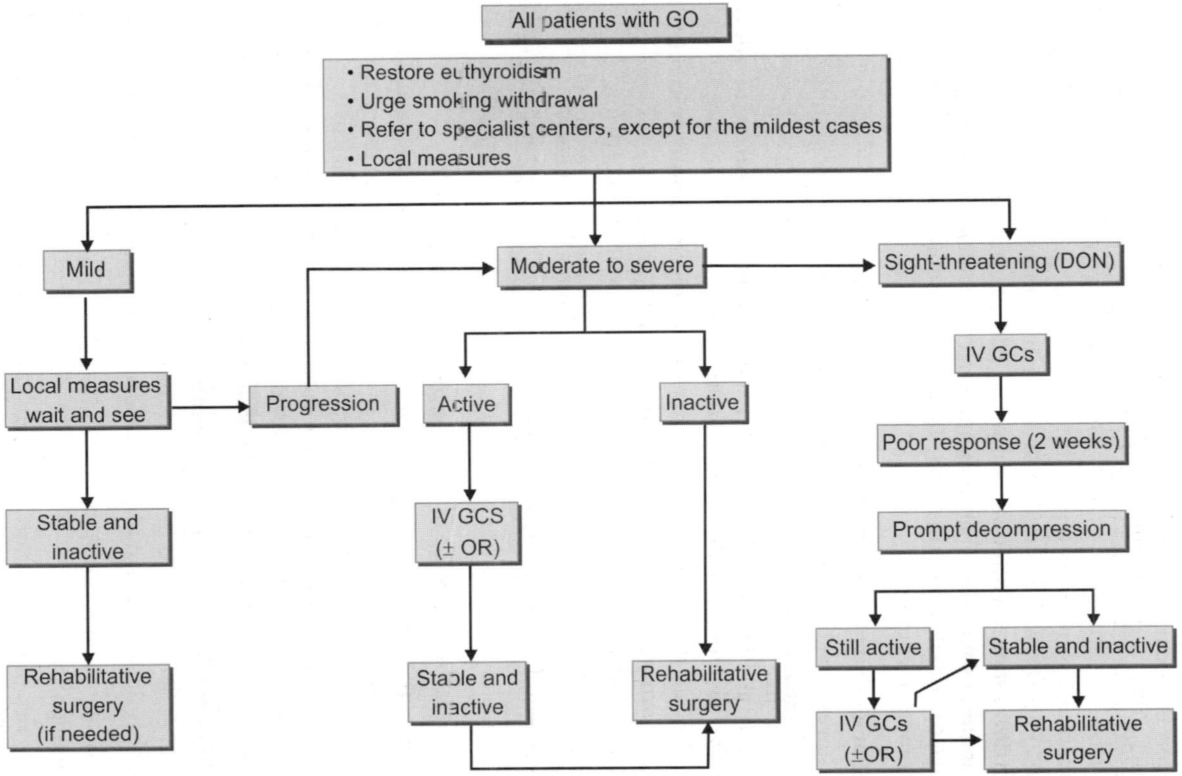

Source: Consensus statement of the European Group on Graves' orbitopathy (EUGOGO) on management of GO. European Journal of Endocrinology. 2008;158:273-85

Q. 6 What are the other options available for patients who do not respond to glucocorticoids?

Ans. Azathioprine, somatostatin analogs, IV immunoglobulin, rituximab have been tried with minimal proven value.

Q. 7 How is moderate-severe ophthalmopathy, i.e. inactive managed?

Ans. Once the disease is inactive, management is specific to the nature of complaints. Patients with exophthalmos benefit from orbital decompression. It is important to reassess and verify, if the disease is inactive before planning surgery. Patients with restriction of ocular movements leading to squint may benefit from squint correction surgeries. Patients may also benefit from lid lengthening procedures. If there is one patient requiring all three procedures, then decompression is done first, followed by squint surgery and then lid lengthening, if required.

Q. 8 How should mild ophthalmopathy be managed?

Ans. Graves' ophthalmopathy is a self-limiting disease hence in mild ophthalmopathy, watchful waiting is a reasonable treatment plan.

Q. 9 What are the simple measures that can be undertaken to alleviate discomfort in patients with ophthalmopathy?

Ans. Lubricant eye drops during the day and lubricant ointments in the night will relieve symptoms of grittiness due to corneal exposure.

Head end elevation by 30° at night can reduce swelling and edema.

Use of protective eye wear, tinted may be encouraged to reduce discomfort while outdoors.

Symptomatic diplopia can be dealt with use of prisms alone.

Lid retraction can be improved with local botulinum toxin injections.

Q. 10 What is the relevance of smoking to ophthalmopathy?

Ans. There is a strong and consistent association between smoking and Graves' orbitopathy (GO). A dose–response relationship between the numbers of cigarettes smoked per day and the probability of developing GO exists.

Smoking also delays or worsens the outcomes of treatments for GO.

Hence, every patient needs to be counseled about the need to quit smoking and seek help from de-addiction experts, if needed.

Q. 11 Does the thyroid status affect ophthalmopathy?

Ans. Every attempt should be made to restore euthyroid status as both a state of hyperthyroidism and hypothyroidism can be detrimental to ophthalmopathy.

Q. 12 What is the position of radioiodine therapy in patients with ophthalmopathy?

Ans. The risk of exacerbation of pre-existing GO following radioiodine therapy is negligible, especially in patients with inactive ophthalmopathy, as long as postradioiodine hypothyroidism is avoided. A definite proportion of patients, especially patients with active disease experience the progression of pre-existing GO within 6 months after radioiodine therapy.

This risk is almost eliminated by giving a short course (4–12 weeks) of oral glucocorticoids after radioiodine therapy, and avoiding post-treatment hypothyroidism.

Our patient is given a course of oral steroids for 4–6 weeks for his ophthalmopathy and he is also started on methimazole in divided doses. He is strictly instructed to stop smoking. He is instructed about eye care and lubrication. At review, his diplopia has improved and the clinical activity score is down to 1/7 both eyes. The dose of methimazole is reduced and the dose of steroid tapered down gradually over 3 weeks.

SUGGESTED READING

1. American Thyroid Association Guidelines for Diagnosis and Management of Hyperthyroidism and Other Causes of Thyrotoxicosis. THYROID. 2016;26:10.
2. Consensus statement of the European Group on Graves' orbitopathy (EUGOGO) on management of GO. European Journal of Endocrinology. 2008;158:273-85.
3. The American Thyroid Association Taskforce on Thyroid Disease During Pregnancy and Postpartum. Thyroid. 2011;21(10):1081-125.
4. Werner and Ingbar's Thyroid: A Fundamental and Clinical Text, 10th edn. Lippincott Williams and Wilkins, 2012.

CHAPTER

8

Approach to Thyroid Nodule

Pramila Kalra

CASE 1

A 26-year-old lady presents with an incidentally noticed swelling in the right side of the neck region which she noticed about 2 weeks back. She had not noticed the swelling earlier.

She is concerned about whether this could be malignant.

The size of the swelling is 20 mm × 20 mm.

There are no compressive symptoms such as change in voice, swallowing difficulty or difficulty in breathing.

She has no history suggestive of hyperthyroidism or hypothyroidism.

There is no family history of any thyroid disorder or any thyroid cancer.

She has no history of any radiation exposure to the neck in the past.

She does not belong to an iodine deficient area.

She is getting married in next 2 months but wants to clear any doubts about the swelling.

What is the next course of action for her?

She is advised to go for thyroid function tests to check for any evidence of hyperthyroidism or hypothyroidism.

Her TSH is 2 mIU/L

And her T4 is 9 ug/dL

T3 is 87 ng/mL

Anti-TPO is 42 U/L

Should she be subjected to surgery?

Should she be asked to go for any further tests?

Q. 1 What are the different types of thyroid nodules?

Ans. Thyroid nodules are extremely common. An estimated prevalence of palpable thyroid nodules is approximately 5% in women and 1% in men in iodine sufficient world. In contrast, high-resolution ultrasound (US) can detect thyroid nodules in 19–68% of randomly selected individuals with higher frequencies in women and the elderly people. With the frequent use of computed tomographic scans and carotid ultrasound studies, many thyroid nodules are found in asymptomatic patients.

Q. 2 What is the fine-needle aspiration cytology (FNAC) classification of thyroid nodule as per the Bethesda system?

Ans.

Bethesda diagnostic category	
I	Non-diagnostic or unsatisfactory
II	Benign
III	Atypia of undetermined significance or follicular lesion of undetermined significance
IV	Follicular neoplasm or suspicious for a follicular neoplasm
V	Suspicious for malignancy
VI	Malignant

Q. 3 What is the biochemical evaluation for such patients?

Ans. According to ATA guidelines, serum TSH should be measured during the initial evaluation of a patient with thyroid nodule. If the serum TSH is low, a radionuclide thyroid scan should be performed. If the serum TSH is normal or elevated, radionuclide thyroid scan should not be performed as the initial imaging evaluation. Serum thyroglobulin (Tg) for initial evaluation is not recommended.

Q. 4 What points should be asked in history?

Ans. The patients should be asked about family history of benign or malignant thyroid disease and familial medullary thyroid carcinoma (MTC), multiple endocrine neoplasia type 2 (MEN 2), familial papillary thyroid tumors, familial polyposis coli, Cowden's disease, and Gardner's syndrome.

Q. 5 What are the causes of thyroid nodules?

Ans. The causes include benign nodular goiter, chronic lymphocytic thyroiditis, simple or hemorrhagic cysts, follicular adenomas, subacute thyroiditis, papillary carcinoma, follicular carcinoma, Hürthle cell carcinoma, poorly differentiated carcinoma, medullary carcinoma, anaplastic carcinoma, primary thyroid lymphoma, sarcoma, teratoma, and miscellaneous tumor and metastatic tumors.

Q. 6 What are the pointers towards malignancy?

Ans. The features which suggest malignancy are history of head and neck irradiation, family history of medullary thyroid carcinoma, multiple endocrine neoplasia type 2, or papillary thyroid carcinoma, age <14 or >70 years, male sex, growing nodule, firm or hard consistency, cervical adenopathy, fixed nodule, persistent dysphonia, dysphagia, or dyspnea.

Q. 7 What type of ultrasound is to be performed?

Ans. High-resolution ultrasound (US) is the most sensitive test available to detect thyroid lesions, measure their dimensions, identify their structure, and evaluate diffuse changes in the thyroid gland.

If results of palpation are normal, US should be performed when a thyroid disorder is suspected on clinical grounds, or if risk factors have been recognized.

The physical finding of suspicious neck adenopathy warrants US examination of both lymph nodes and thyroid gland because of the risk of a metastatic lesion from an otherwise unrecognized papillary microcarcinoma.

Q. 8 When do we need to do fine needle aspiration (FNA) biopsy of thyroid nodules?

Ans. About 50% of thyroid glands with a "solitary" nodule on the basis of palpation have other small nodules which are discovered by US. For MNGs, the cytologic sampling should be focused on lesions with suspicious US features rather than on larger or clinically dominant nodules.

Q. 9 What is the US and color Doppler features which can predict malignancy in a thyroid nodule?

Ans. The reported specificities for predicting malignancy are 41.4–92.2% for marked hypoechogenicity, 44.2–95.0% for microcalcifications (small, intranodular, punctate, hyperechoic spots with scanty or no posterior acoustic shadowing), 48.3–91.8% for irregular or microlobulated margins, and about 80% for chaotic arrangement or intranodular vascular images. The value of these features for predicting cancer is partially blunted by the low sensitivities, however, and no US sign independently is fully predictive of a malignant lesion. A rounded appearance or a "more tall (anteroposterior) than wide (transverse)" shape of the nodule is an additional US pattern suggestive of malignant potential. The coexistence of 2 or more suspicious US criteria greatly increases the risk of thyroid cancer.

Q. 10 What type of physical features need to be noted on examination?

Ans. A careful physical examination to note the size of the nodule location, consistency, adenopathy and any evidence of neck tenderness to be noted.

A single dominant or solitary nodule is more likely to represent carcinoma than a single nodule within a multinodular gland, with an incidence of malignancy from 2.7% to 30% and 1.4% to 10%, respectively. However, the overall risk of malignancy within a gland with a solitary nodule is approximately equal to that of a multinodular gland due to the additive risk of each nodule.

Q. 11 What is management guideline?

Ans. A thyroid nodule is a discrete lesion within the thyroid gland that is radiologically distinct from the surrounding thyroid parenchyma. Generally, only nodules >1 cm should be evaluated, since they have a greater potential to be clinically significant cancers. Occasionally, there may be nodules <1 cm that require evaluation because of suspicious US findings, if it is associated with lymphadenopathy, or other high-risk clinical factors.

Q. 12 What is the prevalence of nodules?

Ans. The estimated prevalence on the basis of palpation ranges from 3% to 7%. The prevalence of clinically unapparent thyroid nodules is estimated in US at 20–76% in the general population, with a prevalence similar to that reported from autopsy data. Moreover, 20–48% of patients with one palpable thyroid nodule are found to have additional nodules on US investigation.

Q. 13 What are the USG features which suggest malignancy?

Ans. A thyroid nodule with firm or hard consistency is associated with high risk of malignancy, high resolution thyroid ultrasound is the most sensitive test for thyroid nodules, internal content of the nodule, microcalcification, margins shape—a taller than wide shape is also suggestive of malignancy, echogenicity—hypoechogenicity is a typical feature of thyroid cancer vascularity—intranodal and chaotic vascularity as one single feature may not be the criteria to diagnose malignancy. A combination of these features points towards a diagnosis of malignancy.

Elastography is very sensitive and specific for the diagnosis of malignancy

Thyroid nodule size is not a predictor factor for malignancy.

Most guidelines recommend FNA for nodules larger than 10 mm.

Q. 14 What are the high risk factors?

Ans. The high-risk factors include a history of thyroid cancer in one or more first-degree relatives, a history of exposure to external beam radiation or ionizing radiation in childhood or adolescence, prior hemithyroidectomy with discovery of thyroid cancer, fluorodeoxyglucose (^{18}F) avidity on positron-emission tomography scanning, multiple endocrine neoplasia (MEN) 2/familial medullary thyroid cancer-associated RET proto-oncogene mutation, or calcitonin levels >100 pg/mL.

Focal [^{18}F] fluorodeoxyglucose positron emission tomography (^{18}FDG-PET) uptake within a sonographically confirmed thyroid nodule conveys an increased risk of thyroid cancer, and FNA is recommended for those nodules ≥1 cm.

Diffuse ^{18}FDG-PET uptake, in conjunction with sonographic and clinical evidence of chronic lymphocytic thyroiditis, does not require further imaging or FNA.

FDG-PET/CT does not play a role in the workup of a nodule but any ^{18}FDG-avid thyroid nodule found incidentally deserves a thorough workup for malignancy.

Q. 15 What is the rate of detection of nodules?

Ans. The overall incidence of thyroid cancer is about 9.2–13% in patients with thyroid nodules who undergo FNA. Also, the high detection rate of US makes FNA for all US-detected nodules impractical, if not impossible. Therefore, deciding which nodules should be biopsied is an important medical issue to ensure that no clinically significant thyroid cancers are missed.

Q. 16 What are the criteria to decide interval growth?

Ans. Nodule growth is defined when a nodule shows more than a 50% increase in volume or a 20% increase in at least two nodule dimensions with a minimal increase of 2 mm in solid or in the solid portion of mixed nodules in order to minimize interobserver bias of each measurement.

Q. 17 How frequently a benign thyroid nodule needs to followed up with ultrasound and FNAC?

Ans. A repeat ultrasonography needs to be done at 1 year, and if there is no change in the size of the nodule at one year then a repeat USG at 3–5 years is needed.

The above patient undergoes an FNAC of the thyroid nodule which shows a colloid nodular goiter. She is asked to follow-up at 6 months with a repeat ultrasound of the thyroid which shows no change in the size of the nodule, and henceforth she is asked to follow-up once in a year with an ultrasound.

Q. 18 What are the different types of thyroid nodule?

Ans. Depending on the components of the internal part of the thyroid nodule, nodules can be classified into cystic, mixed (both solid and cystic components), and solid nodules. In cases where microcysts are aggregated in mixed nodules, the nodule is further defined as spongiform anechoic cyst is definitely benign and can contain hyperechoic spots with comet tail artifacts. The comet tail artifacts are related to microcrystals inside colloid cysts which should be differentiated from the microcalcifications of malignant nodules. Solidity itself is not considered a suspicious US feature. However, several guidelines recommend FNA in solid nodules larger than 10 mm and mixed echoic nodules larger than 15 mm.

CASE 2

- A 42-year-old male with no active medical problem noticed a thyroid nodule 1 year back and was told by ENT specialist not to worry about it. Now he has come as he feels that the nodule is becoming more prominent.
- *Physical examination:* 1 × 2 cm right lower pole nodule. There is also a lymph node which is hard and about 2 cm in size in the upper cervical chain in the right lateral neck region.

  An ultrasound is done which shows features of multinodular goiter. The FNA is done from the lymph node which showed metastatic papillary thyroid cancer.

  The patient was subjected to total thyroidectomy with radical neck dissection.

Q. 1 What is the gender predominance of thyroid nodule?

Ans. Thyroid nodules are more common in women than men by a ratio of 4 to 1. However, the mortality rates are higher in men with thyroid cancer probably because of the older age at diagnosis in men.

Q. 2 What are the other risk factors?

Ans.

- Radiation to head and neck.
  - 40% risk of thyroid cancer usually 25 years later.
  - Exposed populations—Polynesian studies
- Iodine deficiency
- Family history of MEN II, Gardner's syndrome, Cowden's disease.

Q. 3 What are the pointers in history to a malignant change?

Ans. Recent growth, soft tissue swelling, vocal changes, dysphagia.

Q. 4 How should examination of thyroid be carried out?

Ans.

- Use both hands simultaneously to evaluate for symmetry
- Patient should be upright for screening examination
- Patient supine with neck in extension for detailed exam. Swallowing assists in elevating gland
- Evaluation of other neck structures
- Voice changes (recurrent laryngeal nerve).

Q. 5 What is the sensitivity and specificity of fine-needle aspiration cytology?

Ans.

- Best tool for determining pathology other than surgical excision
- Can be as high as 80% sensitive and 95% specific
- Operator dependent in obtaining adequate amount of tissue. 25-gauge needle is optimal
- Should not be relied on if negative in patient with previous neck irradiation—multifocal tumors are common.

Q. 6 How do we interpret the biopsy reports?

Ans. Benign, indeterminate, suspicious, inadequate specimen.

Q. 7 What do these terms mean?

Ans.

- *Benign:* 90–95% likelihood, it is benign
- *Indeterminate:* Who knows?
- *Suspicious:* It is malignant.
- *Inadequate specimen:* Do it again (and again).

Q. 8 What is US elastography?

Ans. US elastography (USE) is a recent technological advance that measures tissue elasticity or stiffness properties objectively and has been available in recent years on many state-of-the-art clinical US machines. USE is classified as diagnostic ultrasound and is safe, noninvasive and requires no costly consumables. Importantly, USE can be performed in real-time alongside conventional sonography, providing objective stiffness data that can be used to influence clinical decisions during US examinations. The clinical potential of USE relies on the same principles as clinical palpation, namely that processes such as malignancy and fibrosis alter elasticity.

Q. 9 When to perform thyroid ultrasound?

Ans. Patients who should be subjected to thyroid ultrasound include those at risk for malignancy, solitary nodule or multinodular goiter, patients with lymphadenopathy which is suspicious of malignancy.

Q. 10 Whether in the above patient the lymph node or the nodule should have been biopsied?

Ans. For patients without a high-risk history, one should look for abnormal cervical lymph nodes if present, detected by either physical examination or ultrasound study. If so, biopsy samples should be obtained from the lymph nodes themselves, with or without biopsy of any suspicious thyroid nodules present. In the above-mentioned patient, biopsy sample is collected from the lymph node which shows metastatic thyroid cancer.

Q. 11 What is the advantage of MRI or CT scan for diagnosis of malignant thyroid nodule?

Ans. MRI or CT are not useful for the diagnosis of thyroid nodule except in very advanced cases.

Q. 12 Which nodules are suitable for FNAC?

Ans. The nodules which should be subjected to FNAC include nodules of diameter larger than 1 cm which are solid and hypoechoic on ultrasound or coexistence of 2 or more ultrasound features of malignancy, any size of the nodule with extracapsular growth or metastatic cervical lymph node, history of chest and neck irradiation in childhood, any nodule with features of high risk for malignancy. Hot nodules on scintigraphy can be excluded from FNAC.

Q. 13 What should be done for a multinodular goiter?

Ans. Patients with multiple thyroid nodules ≥1 cm should be evaluated in the same fashion as patients with a solitary nodule ≥1 cm, excepting that each nodule that is >1 cm carries an independent risk of malignancy and therefore multiple nodules may require FNA. When multiple nodules ≥1 cm are present, FNA should be performed preferentially based upon nodule sonographic pattern and respective size cutoff.

Q. 14 Is large needle and core needle biopsy recommended for thyroid nodule?

Ans. It is not recommended because of the pain associated with it and the risk of hemorrhage. It also does not add anything to the diagnosis.

Q. 15 Should calcitonin levels be measured in all patients with thyroid nodule?

Ans. It is necessary in those patients with a suspicion of medullary thyroid cancer or with a family history of MEN or medullary thyroid cancer. It should be measured in those patients with a FNA diagnosis of medullary thyroid cancer or with a nodular goiter who are planned for surgery to avoid risk of incomplete removal or inadequate surgery.

Q. 16 The TSH of the patient discussed above is normal. Should we do further biochemical evaluation?

Ans. The recommendation is to do free thyroxine and anti-TPO antibodies, if the TSH level is increased. The TSH receptor antibody should be done, if the TSH is suppressed. The need to do thyroglobulin antibody is only in those patients where there is a suspicion of chronic lymphocytic thyroiditis and serum levels of anti-TPO are normal. The routine measurement of serum thyroglobulin as initial assessment is not recommended in all patients with thyroid nodule.

Q. 17 Is there any role of thyroid scintigraphy in this patient?

Ans. Serum TSH should be measured during the initial evaluation of a patient with a thyroid nodule. If the serum TSH is subnormal, a radionuclide (preferably ^{123}I) thyroid scan should be performed. If the serum TSH is normal or elevated, then a radionuclide scan should not be performed as the initial imaging evaluation. Radionuclide scan can be done with TC99m Pertechnetate also in place of ^{123}I.

Q. 18 What is TIRADS?

Ans. It is thyroid imaging reporting and data system. It is done by ultrasonography.

TIRADS 1: Normal thyroid gland

TIRADS 2: Benign lesions, score zero

TIRADS 3: Probably benign lesions (<5% risk of malignancy), score zero

TIRADS 4

- 4a: Undetermined nodules (5–10% risk of malignancy), Score of 1
- 4b: Suspicious nodules (10–50% risk of malignancy), Score of 2
- 4c: Highly suspicious nodules (50–85% risk of malignancy), Score of 3–4

TIRADS 5: Probably malignant nodules (>85% risk of malignancy) Score of 5 or higher

TIRADS 6: Biopsy proven malignancy.

Q. 19 What is the strategy for sonographic follow-up of these nodules based upon nodule sonographic pattern?

Ans.

- Nodules with high suspicion US pattern: repeat US in 6–12 months.
- Nodules with sonographic features of low-to-intermediate suspicion US pattern: consider repeat US at 12–24 months.
- Nodules >1 cm with very low suspicion US pattern (including spongiform nodules) and pure cyst: the utility and time interval of surveillance US for risk of malignancy is not known. If US is repeated, it should be at >24 months.
- Nodules <1 cm with very low suspicion US pattern (including spongiform nodules) and pure cysts do not require routine sonographic follow-up.
- Nodules <5 mm without high suspicion US pattern do not require routine sonographic FU and if repeated, the US should be performed at 24 months or later.

Q. 20 How to manage a case of FNA proven thyroid malignancy?

Ans. The basic goal of treatment is to improve overall survival, reduce the risk of recurrent disease and associated morbidity, and permit accurate disease staging and risk stratification, while minimizing treatment-related morbidity and unnecessary therapy. Surgical intervention is the treatment of choice.

SUGGESTED READING

1. Giannini R, Torregrossa L, Gottardi S, Fregoli L, Borrelli N, Savino M, et al. Digital gene expression profiling of a series of cytologically indeterminate thyroid nodules. Cancer Cytopathol, 2015. doi: 10.1002/cncy.21564. [Epub ahead of print]

2. Ha EJ, Baek JH, Kim KW, Pyo J, Lee JH, Baek SH, et al. Comparative efficacy of radiofrequency and laser ablation for the treatment of benign thyroid nodules: systematic review including traditional pooling and bayesian network meta-analysis. J Clin Endocrinol Metab. 2015;100(5):1903-11.
3. Haugen BR, Alexander EK, Bible KC, Doherty GM, Mandel SJ, Nikiforov YE, et al. 2015 American Thyroid Association Management Guidelines for Adult Patients with Thyroid Nodules and Differentiated Thyroid Cancer: The American Thyroid Association Guidelines Task Force on Thyroid Nodules and differentiated Thyroid Cancer. Thyroid. 2016;26(1):1-133.
4. Jung CK, Min HS, Park HJ, Song DE, Kim JH, Park SY, et al. Korean Endocrine Pathology Thyroid Core Needle Bio. Pathology Reporting of Thyroid Core Needle Biopsy: A Proposal of the Korean Endocrine Pathology Thyroid Core Needle Biopsy Study Group. J Pathol Transl Med; 2015. doi:10.4132/jptm.2015.06.04. [Epub ahead of print].
5. Kim JY, Jung SL, Kim MK, Kim TJ, Byun JY. Differentiation of benign and malignant thyroid nodules based on the proportion of sponge-like areas on ultrasonography: imaging-pathologic correlation. Ultrasonography; 2015. doi: 10.14366/usg.15016. [Epub ahead of print].
6. Kist JW, Nell S, de Keizer B, Valk GD, Borel Rinkes IH, Vriens MR. The role of qualitative elastography in thyroid nodule evaluation: exploring its target populations. Endocrine; 2015.
7. Lsayed NM, Elkhatib YA. Diagnostic Criteria and Accuracy of Malignant Thyroid Nodules by Ultrasonography and Ultrasound Elastography with Pathologic Correlation. Ultrason Imaging; 2015. pii: 0161734615584906. [Epub ahead of print]
8. Yoon JH, Lee HS, Kim EK, Moon HJ, Kwak JY. Thyroid Nodules: Nondiagnostic Cytologic Results according to Thyroid Imaging Reporting and Data System before and after Application of the Bethesda System. Radiology; 2015:142308. [Epub ahead of print].

CHAPTER

9

Approach to Sick Euthyroid Syndrome or Nonthyroidal Illness Syndrome

Pramila Kalra

CASE 1

A 38-year-old female with no previous history of any thyroid problem is admitted in the ICU with septic shock.

> Avoid doing TFT in a sick patient unless indicated.

Patient is on ventilator for past 3 days and has thyroid profile as below:

- T3–66 ng/dL (75–200 ng/dL)
- T4–3 µg/dL (4.5–11.5 µg/dL)
- TSH 0.2 µIU/L (0.45–4.5 µIU/L)

A consultation is sent to endocrinology department for treatment of probable hypothyroidism?

What is the interpretation of these results?

The patient's differential diagnosis could be:

- Secondary hypothyroidism
- Sick euthyroid syndrome or nonthyroid illness syndrome (NTIS)

The diagnosis of sick euthyroid syndrome is kept as the first possibility in this case because she has no prior history of thyroid problem and has no history of being treated for hypothyroidism in the past.

> Prior history of deranged TFT can be helpful in reaching a diagnosis.

The secondary hypothyroidism is also kept as a possibility so to evaluate for any other pituitary hormone deficiency a random serum cortisol is done along with prolactin, FSH and LH. There is no prior history of pituitary problem in this patient.

The FT4 and FT3 are also ordered in this patient.

The patient's FT4 is 1 ng/L (0.8–2 ng/L) and FT3 is 2 pg/mL (2.3–4.2 pg/mL).

The serum cortisol is elevated and it is 52 µg/dL because of the stress state and during severe stress serum cortisol can be more than 50 µg/dL and it should be at least more than 25 μg/dL and prolactin is also in the high normal range (36 ng/mL) which is also probably a stress response. Rest of the pituitary hormones are in the normal range.

The patient was normally menstruating till the last month so it was also an indirect evidence that the gonadotropic axis is intact.

The patient improves over a period of time in the next 2 weeks and thyroid profile is repeated after 2 weeks where it shows the following results:

- FT4—1.2 ng/mL
- T4—5 ug/dL
- T3—78 ng/dL
- TSH—5.6 μ IU/mL

Q. 1 What is nonthyroidal illness syndrome or NTIS?

Ans. The nonthyroidal illness syndrome (NTIS) is defined as low T3 syndrome or sick euthyroid syndrome and is a very common entity seen in wide variety of critical illnesses and acute and chronic stress conditions. Critical illness is defined as a life-threatening condition where support is needed for function of vital organs. NTIS was first reported in 1970 and it affects about 70% of hospitalized patients.

'Nonthyroidal illness syndrome' (NTIS) is now more commonly used for such changes in thyroid related hormones which are not due to inherent abnormality of the thyroid function.

Q. 2 What are the reasons for changes in the thyroid hormones during illness?

Ans. These changes were initially thought of as a compensatory response of the body to fight the stress state but now new insights have come into the pathophysiology of the syndrome. The laboratory parameters of this syndrome include low serum levels of triiodothyronine (T3) and high levels of reverse T3 (rT3), with normal or low levels of thyroxine (T4) and normal or low levels of thyroid-stimulating hormone (TSH). The reverse T3 may be normal in some cases and it may be inhibited by low level of T4 in the blood. There is a blunted response of TSH to the stimulation by TRH (thyrotropin releasing hormone). About 3% of the patients may have TSH value lower than 0.1 mIU/mL and out of these 75% of these cases may have NTIS.

Q. 3 Is there alteration in the levels of the other hormones also along with thyroid hormones?

Ans. There are alterations in other hormone levels along with the abnormalities in thyroid hormones. The levels of gonadotropin decrease, while the levels of ACTH and cortisol rise, so the changes in the thyroid hormone levels could be viewed as part of endocrine hormone alteration in critical illness.

These patients generally do not need thyroid hormone replacement therapy but the level of the thyroid hormone may be a prognostic marker and low levels of the hormones have been found to be associated with increased mortality.

Q. 4 What is the pathogenesis?

Ans. There are multiple mechanisms behind the pathophysiology of NTIS. NTIS results from changes in the transcription and translation of genes involved in thyroid hormone metabolism which may result in stimulation or inhibition of the gene depending on the tissue studied and also alteration in thyroid hormone deiodinating enzymes (D1, D2 and D3) in various tissues. Granulocyte is a major cell involved in NTIS during bacterial infection. Medications may also be the incriminating agents.

Q. 5 What changes occur in the level of thyroid hormones?

Ans. The initial changes seen in the thyroid function tests include decrease in the T3 levels. The levels of reverse T3 (rT3) are usually elevated. Elevation of rT3 was initially thought of as a differentiation marker from hypothyroidism but further studies have not corroborated the same. As the illness progresses fall in the levels of T4 and TSH also occurs. FT4 levels are generally in the normal range but may become low or slightly increased depending on the underlying disease.

Q. 6 What is the change in the circadian rhythm of TSH secretion in patients with NTIS?

Ans. The TSH secretion follows a circadian rhythm with peak secretion between 9 pm and 5 am and a minimum secretion between 4 pm and 7 pm but in patients with NTIS the normal nocturnal surge of TSH is decreased or is entirely absent

Q. 7 What is the pathophysiology of sick euthyroid syndrome?

Ans. It is postulated that in sick euthyroid syndrome inhibition of 5'-deiodinase enzyme is the main mechanism. The initial pathophysiology is acute inhibition of the enzyme type 1, 5'-deiodinase which leads to decreased conversion of T4 to T3 in extrathyroidal tissue. The sick state causes a reduced activity of 5' monodeiodinases and increase in the activity of 5' deiodinase which results in reduced conversion of T4 to T3 and increased conversion of T4 to rT3 which is also called the inactivating pathway. The changes in serum FT3 and FT4 may be modest compared to the changes seen in the levels of T3 and T4. The deiodination of inner ring T4 is not affected at all so the concentration of reverse T3 increases while the breakdown of rT3 is decreased as the type 1, 5'-deiodinase is inhibited during acute illness. It has been shown in knockout mice that the fall of T3 in sick state may occur independently of the DI and D2 enzymes and the fall in T3 levels precede the onset of hepatic D1 inhibition. The thyrotropin levels decrease possibly secondary to decrease in leptin caused by malnutrition and there is a localized increase in hypothalamic T3 catalyzed by altered expression of hypothalamic iodothyronine deiodinases D2 and D3. 5'-deiodinase converts rT3 to T2 and its reduced activity slows the clearance of rT3 and thus its level rises in the blood.

Deiodinases play a role in thyroid hormone metabolism not only in the periphery but also in the hypothalamus and the pituitary and thus in the alterations accompanying NTIS.

Q. 8 Is there any role of cytokines in the pathogenesis of sick euthyroid syndrome?

Ans. The cytokines, released during illness, are known to affect a variety of genes involved in TH metabolism and are therefore considered a major determinant.

There are numerous inflammatory cytokines or other inflammatory mediators like tumor necrosis factor, interferon-alpha, NF-κB and interleukin-6 and interleukin-10 which are incriminated in the etiopathogenesis of NTIS.

CASE 2

A 5-year-old male child is admitted post valvular surgery to cardiac ICU.

A consultation is sent saying that there is a suspicion of secondary hypothyroidism.

The results are as below

- T3–80 ng/dL (94–269 ng/dL)
- T4–3 μg/dL (7–15 μg/dL)
- TSH–0.02 μ IU/mL (0.5–5.0 μ IU/L)

What is the clinical diagnosis in this case?

What is the next step in evaluation of this patient?

What other parameters can help in the diagnosis?

The child was evaluated for other evidences of hypopituitarism as below

The child is in the 5th centile which is expected as the child had untreated cyanotic congenital heart disease because of which the growth is stunted so probably growth hormone deficiency does not exist.

The child has no evidence of micropenis so hypopituitarism was less of a possibility as it can be a marker of hypopituitarism.

The child is maintaining blood pressure and is not requiring any ionotropic support which is an indirect evidence of normal cortisol levels.

Thus, the clinical diagnosis in this child is kept as sick euthyroid syndrome as the other pituitary hormones are normal and there is no clinical evidence of hypopituitarism in this child.

The levels of FT4 and FT3 are also done and FT4 is found to be in the normal range for age while FT3 is low.

The other anterior pituitary hormones including random serum cortisol, FSH, LH and prolactin are measured in this child and the levels are found to be normal as per the clinical state of the patient. An IGF-1 level is done to screen for growth hormone deficiency and it is found to be in the normal range for age and sex matched controls.

Different critical illness states leading to NTIS

- Sepsis and trauma
- Starvation
- Cardiac dysfunction
- Renal disease
- Hepatic disease
- Nonseptic shock
- Burns
- Respiratory failure
- Other disease states like systemic sclerosis

Q. 1 How to diagnose a case of NTIS?

Ans. The diagnosis of sick euthyroid syndrome is very challenging. History may not provide any clue to the diagnosis of nonthyroidal illness syndrome (NTIS), only there may not be any past history of any thyroid illness and the recent illness may be severe enough to cause NTIS.

The physical examination is mostly unremarkable. There may be masking of hypothyroidism or hyperthyroidism in such cases. The thyroid gland examination is mostly normal. The patient will mostly have signs of the illness he is having.

The two general principles which should be kept in mind while evaluating thyroid function in a sick patient are that the thyroid functions should be done only if there is a strong suspicion of thyroid disease and the full thyroid profile is mostly necessary for proper interpretation of results.

Within hours after the illness the level of T3 decrease while the level of T4 and TSH may increases slightly.

If any patient has a low TSH value then if the T3 is low it may go in favor of sick euthyroid syndrome and if the T3 is high it is suggestive of hyperthyroidism.

Some patients who are very sick may have low T3 value even with hyperthyroidism. The measurement of FT4 as it may mostly be in the normal range in normal patients even in the sick state except in cases where the patient is very sick where even FT4 may decrease. In most cases of hyperthyroidism TSH is suppressed to less than 0.01mIU/mL but in cases of NTIS it is mostly more than 0.01 mIU/mL.

In the recovery phase the level of TSH mostly reaches up to 20 mIU/mL but in about 3% cases it may even reach up to 30 mIU/mL. The levels of TSH more than 30 mIU/mL mostly favors a diagnosis of primary hypothyroidism.

The cases of secondary hypothyroidism may be difficult to differentiate from nonthyroidal illness as both will show low TSH, T4 and T3 values but measurement of rT3 may provide some guidance though it has also not been shown to be a very accurate tool for differentiation. The measurement of prolactin, serum gonadotropin, stimulated cortisol may be of help in such cases where differentiation from secondary hypothyroidism is difficult. The low levels of other pituitary hormones may be an indicator of pituitary deficiency and may thus suggest secondary hypothyroidism.

In some cases differentiation from hyperthyroidism is difficult as these patients may present with suppressed TSH with a normal value of T3 and T4 because of the coexistent catabolic state or infection. The levels of thyroxine-blinding globulin (TBG) may be decrease in such cases which may give a lower value of total T4 and T3, thus measurement of FT4 may be more useful in such cases as elevated FT4 with undetectable or suppressed TSH may confirm the diagnosis of hyperthyroidism.

Any previous history of thyroid disorder, presence of goiter, history of irradiation to the neck or a surgical scar suggesting previous thyroidectomy may point towards a primary thyroid disorder.

Thyroid imaging may provide some clue to the correct diagnosis.

Q. 2 Do these patients benefit from hormone supplementation?

Ans. Treatment with thyroid hormone is controversial. The studies done so far have not conclusive benefit with levothyroxine replacement therapy in patients with sick euthyroid syndrome. Intravenous T3 administration is preferred as the peripheral conversion of T4 to T3 is decreased due to the reduced activity of 5'deiodinase enzyme.

Moreover, the use of thyroxine in patients with sick euthyroid syndrome may induce subclinical hyperthyroidism and T3 administration may exert negative effect on protein and fat metabolism and causes a rise in catecholamine levels.

Thus the use of T3 in patients with NTIS and cardiac disease remains controversial.

In some studies intravenous infusion of T3 has not shown any mortality benefit while in few it has been shown that after elective coronary artery bypass grafting the need of ionotropic support, incidence of postoperative myocardial ischemia and need of mechanical ventilation was reduced in patients who were given triiodothyronine.

In acute renal failure and burn patients, thyroid hormone supplementation has not been shown to provide any mortality benefits.

Thyrotropin releasing hormone (TRH) has been tried and has been shown to normalize the thyroid hormone values in a single day in critically ill patients and could be a safer alternative to thyroid hormone supplementation in such patients.

Q. 3 When do the normalization of thyroid hormone level happen?

Ans. The TSH levels normalize during the recovery phase and may even reach up to 20 mIU/mL and may cause a misdiagnosis of primary hypothyroidism as the rise in TSH usually precedes the normalization of T3 and T4 values. This rise in TSH is probably a compensatory phenomenon of the body to bring the T3 and T4 levels to normal range.

The normalization of thyroid hormone levels in sick euthyroid syndrome occurs after 1 month of discharge. Serum TSH at admission has been found to be the only variable negatively correlated to normalization of thyroid function after recovery.

The recovery of thyroid functions after coronary artery bypass grafting has been found to occur within 6 months though some of the patients have been shown to have abnormalities suggestive of NTIS even 6 months after coronary artery by pass grafting.

A continuous infusion of TRH with a growth hormone secretagogue as discussed previously cause a rise of both thyroid hormone and TSH concentration with subsequent improvement in the metabolic parameters in patients with NTIS.

Q. 4 What is the prognostication of NTIS?

Ans. The cumulative illness rating scale (CIRS) scores (severity and comorbidity index) have been found to be inversely related to FT3 and positively related to

FT4 levels and the CRP (C-reactive protein) level is found to be positively associated with FT4 levels.

Serum FT3 values correlates inversely with serum C-reactive protein, lactate dehydrogenase, fibrinogen and erythrocyte sedimentation rate values, and progressively decreased with increasing tertiles of age.

The level of thyroid hormone correlates with mortality. Low T3 is an independent prognostic indicator in cardiac patients. Low T3 syndrome is related to NT-pro-BNP but is an independent predictor of cardiovascular mortality. Determination of rT3 may help in the prognostication of patients who may be at risk of subsequent mortality. The decrease in the level of FT4 over the course of illness has been found to a poor prognostic marker.

The low thyroid hormone is thought of as a better predictor of mortality than APACHE 1 score and has been directly correlated with T4 levels in some studies. A T4 level lower than 4 μg/dL is associated with 50% probability of death while a T4 level lower than 2 μg/dL is associated with 80% probability of death. Reverse T3 to T3 ratio, elevated rT3 are independent predictor of survival. Low T3 and FT4 levels have been found to be adverse prognostic marker.

The patient in case 1 is subsequently followed up in the OPD and thyroid profile becomes normal after 6 weeks of follow-up.

The hormone levels of the child in case 2 becomes normal after four weeks of follow-up without any levothyroxine supplementation and child is discharged in a stable condition from the hospital.

SUGGESTED READING

1. Boelen A, Kwakkel J, Fliers E. Beyond low plasma T3: local thyroid hormone metabolism during inflammation and infection. Endocr Rev. 2011;32(5):670-93. doi: 10.1210/er.2011-0007. Epub 2011 Jul 26. Review.
2. Economidou F, Douka E, Tzanela M, Nanas S, Kotanidou A. Thyroid function during critical illness. Hormones (Athens). 2011;10(2):117-24.
3. Farwell AP. Nonthyroidal illness syndrome. Curr Opin Endocrinol Diabetes Obes. 2013;20(5):478-84.
4. Forceville X. Selenium and the "free" electron. Selenium--a trace to be followed in septic or inflammatory ICU patients? Intensive Care Med. 2001;27(1): 16-8.
5. Lado-Abeal J, Romero A, Castro-Piedras I, Rodriguez-Perez A, Alvarez- Escudero J. Thyroid hormone receptors are down-regulated in skeletal muscle of patientswith non-thyroidal illness syndrome secondary to non-septic shock. Eur JEndocrinol. 2010; 163(5):765-73. Epub 2010 Aug 24.
6. Liu ML, Xu G, Huang ZY, Zhong XC, Liu SH, Jiang TY. Euthyroid sick syndrome and nutritional status are correlated with hyposelenemia in hemodialysis patients. Int J Artif Organs. 2011;34(7):577-83
7. Mebis L, Van den Berghe G. Thyroid axis function and dysfunction in critical illness. Best Pract Res Clin Endocrinol Metab. 2011;25(5):745-57.

8. Meyer S, Schuetz P, Wieland M, Nusbaumer C, Mueller B, Christ-Crain M. Low triiodothyronine syndrome: a prognostic marker for outcome in sepsis? Endocrine. 2011;39(2):167-74. Epub 2011 Jan 6 de.
9. Pappa TA, Vagenakis AG, Alevizaki M. The nonthyroidal illness syndrome in the non-critically ill patient. Eur J Clin Invest. 2011;41(2):212-20. doi:10.1111/j.1365-2362.2010.02395.x. Epub 2010 Oct 21. Review.
10. Vries EM, Fliers E, Boelen A. The molecular basis of the non-thyroidal illness syndrome. J Endocrinol. 2015;225(3):R67-R81. Epub 2015 May 13. Review.
11. Van den Berghe G. Non-thyroidal illness in the ICU: a syndrome with different faces. Thyroid. 2014;24(10):1456-65. doi: 10.1089/thy.2014.0201. Epub 2014 Jun 19. Review.
12. Zeraati AA, Layegh P, Famili Y, Naghibi M, Sharifipour F, Shariati Sarabi Z. Serum triiodothyronine level as an indicator of inflammation in patients undergoing dialysis. Iran J Kidney Dis. 2011;5(1):38-44.

CHAPTER

10

Approach to Gynecomastia

V Sri Nagesh, Altamash Shaikh, KVS Harikumar, Sunil Kota

CASE

A 15-year-old boy presents with history of breast enlargement noticed for the past 3 years. It was initially painful for the first 6 months and subsequently, the pain subsided. At this point, he was evaluated by a pediatrician in his annual school health examination, who noticed small testes in addition to gynecomastia. He was then referred to an endocrinologist for further evaluation, where the boy and his parents give the following clinical history. His birth weight was 3 kg. He was born after a term pregnancy by normal vaginal delivery and had a birth weight of 3 kg. Subsequent postnatal history did not include any neonatal seizures or prolonged neonatal jaundice. Subsequent development was age appropriate. He did not experience any episodes of seizures, or prolonged neonatal jaundice. There was no history of any chronic disease, central nervous system trauma, infections or irradiation. There is no history of abdominal or scrotal trauma, surgery or irradiation. He also did not receive any chemotherapy in the past. He does not give any history suggestive of orchitis or other scrotal infections. There is also no history of anosmia.

His mother, however, complains of below par scholastic performance with average to poor grades. There is no consanguinity, family history of gynecomastia, delayed puberty, anosmia or infertility. Pubertal development was noticed at about 12 years of age. He has one sister who has had normal pubertal development.

On examination, the child has a height of 176 cm and weight of 65 kg. Mid-parental height is 166 cm. Arm span is 184 cm and upper to lower segment ratio was 0.83, which is suggestive of eunuchoid proportions. He has sparse facial hair. Axillary (Tanner Stage 2) and pubic hair (Tanner Stage 3) are sparse but present. Stretched penile length is 7.8 cm and bilaterally testes are palpable, small and firm, with a volume of 5 mL. He does not have goiter. His pulse is 74 per minute, blood pressure is 118/60 mm Hg, and respiratory rate is 18. He has a nontender gynecomastia with 5 cm of palpable tissue on the right and 3 cm on the left.

His abdomen is soft with no palpable masses and other systems are also normal. No anosmia is appreciated on examination.

Biochemical testing reveals normal thyroid, liver and renal functions. Elevated levels of luteinizing hormone (LH) and follicle-stimulating hormone (FSH) at 22 mIU/mL (normal 1.4–12) and 53 mIU/mL (normal 0.6–15 mIU/mL) respectively are discovered, with a low testosterone of 14 ng/dL (normal 350–850 ng/dL). A karyotype is ordered, and is 47XXY, which confirms Klinefelter's syndrome. A detailed evaluation by a psychologist reveals some impulsivity and a normal Intelligence Quotient (IQ).

Q. 1 What is gynecomastia?

Ans. Gynecomastia is defined histologically as a benign proliferation of the glandular tissue of the male breast, and clinically by the presence of a rubbery or firm mass extending concentrically from the nipple. It is a relatively common condition and is usually benign and self-resolving, especially in children. However, it may also be caused by many pathologic conditions. Distinguishing physiological gynecomastia from pathologic gynecomastia is the prime requisite in the management of gynecomastia.

Q. 2 What is physiological gynecomastia?

Ans. Gynecomastia can be commonly seen in neonates, during puberty and in older men. An estimated 60–90% of infants have transient gynecomastia due to transplacental transfer of maternal estrogens. It usually regresses completely by the end of the first year. Around 60% of all boys develop transient pubertal breast enlargement, and 30–70% of adult men have palpable breast tissue, with the higher prevalence being seen in older men and those with concurrent medical illnesses. Gynecomastia may occur in 48–64% of boys at puberty. It may first appear as early as 10 years of age, with a peak onset between ages 13 and 14, followed by a decline in late teenage years. In autopsy studies, histologic evidence of gynecomastia is found in up to half of all men.

Q. 3 What is the pathophysiology of gynecomastia?

Ans. The primary pathophysiology of gynecomastia is an imbalance between the androgens and estrogens. Estrogens stimulate breast tissue growth, whereas androgens inhibit it. This can be caused either by an absolute decrease in testosterone as seen in older men, an increase in estrogens as seen in feminizing tumors and exogenous administration of estrogens, especially throughout the use of oils like lavender oil or tea tree oil, and diethylstilbestrol in prostatic carcinoma. Cases have also resulted from unintended exposure to exogenous estrogens in vaginal creams and hair lotions. An increase in sex hormone binding globulin (SHBG) as is seen in hyperthyroidism can also result in gynecomastia. SHBG binds testosterone more avidly than estrogen, leading to a reduction in free testosterone and androgen to estrogen ratio. Local factors like excessive local production of estrogen due to increased aromatase activity, decreased estrogen degradation, or changes in androgen or estrogen receptors can also contribute to gynecomastia. Hyperprolactinemia does not have a direct role in gynecomastia. However, hyperprolactinemia can indirectly cause gynecomastia by suppressing gonadotropin release and producing secondary hypogonadism, leading to an imbalance in testosterone/estrogen ratio.

Q. 4 What are the local and hormonal factors which can contribute to gynecomastia?

Ans. Increased local production of estrogens due to enhanced aromatase activity in the breast, decreased estrogen inactivation, decreased local production of testosterone from androstenedione, and changes in androgen or estrogen receptors could all contribute to the genesis of gynecomastia. In aging males, there is an increase in adipose tissue. This is coupled with an increase in the aromatase activity of adipose tissue, that can result in a more effective conversion of androgens to estrogens, leading to gynecomastia. Breast tissue also produces numerous growth factors like IGF-1, IGF-2 and epidermal growth factor. The role of these factors in the genesis of gynecomastia is unclear.

Q. 5 What is pseudogynecomastia?

Ans. Pseudogynecomastia is more common in obese adolescents and is commonly mistaken for true gynecomastia. In true gynecomastia, on palpation, firm subareolar tissue can be felt, which is not the case in pseudogynecomastia, where only subcutaneous fat can be felt. These two entities can be differentiated by comparing the subareolar tissue with the anterior axillary fold or other subcutaneous tissue to better appreciate the cord-like palpable breast tissue. Even in true gynecomastia, subcutaneous fat can make even minor gynecomastia seem prominent.

Q. 6 What is the etiology of gynecomastia?

Ans. Gynecomastia has varied etiology and for the sake of simplicity, it can be classified under the following headings:

- Decreased serum androgens
- Increased serum estrogens
- Relative increase in androgen/estrogen ratio.

The various conditions which make up this classification are listed in Box 10.1.

Q. 7 What is refeeding gynecomastia?

Ans. This is an entity which was first reported in the American Prisoners of Wars (POWs) in the Japanese Prison Camps at Bataan in Philippines during the Second World War. A severe lack of prisoner rations led to chronic and sustained underfeeding of the American POWs, which resulted in loss of libido, impotence, generalized decrease in scalp and body hair, spontaneous decrease in acne and seborrheic dermatitis; and some prisoners even claimed to have atrophy of testes, though it could not be proven. After the Japanese surrender and the liberation of these POWs, re-establishment of normal feeding resulted in re-appearance of libido and fertility and almost 300 cases of gynecomastia were reported in these POWs. Almost all of these were tender and bilateral, though breast enlargement on one side preceded enlargement on the other side by a few weeks and a few POWs also reported a colostrum-like breast discharge. Starvation and substantial weight loss are associated with hypogonadotropic hypogonadism, and when nutrition is restored, the hypothalamic-pituitary-testicular axis returns to normal, leading to a situation akin to self-limited puberty gynecomastia. A similar picture

BOX 10.1 Etiology of gynecomastia

Decreased serum androgen production or action
- Primary hypogonadism—Klinefelter's, testicular trauma, tumors and infections, disorders of testicular biosynthesis and action
- Secondary hypogonadism—Kallmann, combined pituitary hormone deficiency, idiopathic hypogonadotropic hypogonadism
- Drugs—spironolactone, ketoconazole, antiandrogens, cancer chemotherapy

Increased serum estrogens
- Feminizing adrenal tumors
- Sertoli cell tumors, Leydig cell tumors
- Exogenous estrogens
- Lavender oil, tea tree oil

Relative decrease in androgen/estrogen ratio
- Refeeding gynecomastia
- Cirrhosis of liver
- Hyperthyroidism
- Post-dialysis gynecomastia
- Puberty
- Aging
- Drugs like aromatase inhibitors

can also be seen after recovery from chronic debilitating illness, in chronic kidney disease patients who manifest recovery after dialysis, in refugees and after therapeutic diets. Gynecomastia in patients on treatment with digoxin or isoniazid could also be due to similar mechanisms, with drug therapy leading to significant improvement in the clinical status and malnutrition.

Q. 8 Is the mechanism in cirrhosis of liver also similar?

Ans. Gynecomastia in cirrhosis of liver operates by multiple mechanisms, including an increase in SHBG levels, causing a decrease in free testosterone, decreased breakdown of androstenedione with a consequent rise in conversion to estrogen, a rise in progesterone which can lead to breast development, and in the case of alcoholic cirrhosis, hypogonadism mediated by alcohol toxicity. However, recent studies have called into question, the commonly held assumption that gynecomastia is more common in people with liver dysfunction when compared to people with normal liver function.

Q. 9 What are the tumors which can cause gynecomastia?

Ans. As mentioned in Box 10.1, various neoplasms constitute a significant minority among the etiology of gynecomastia and are a very important reason why a diligent search should always be made for the cause of gynecomastia, to prevent probable morbidity and mortality. Among the neoplasms which can cause an absolute increase in estrogen levels, the principal ones are testicular Sertoli and Leydig cell tumors. Both are usually benign.

Leydig cell tumors usually occur in the young, though no age is exempt. They secrete estradiol, which causes gynecomastia by three mechanisms. Primarily by absolute excess of estrogen, secondarily by a negative feedback on LH, causing suppression of testosterone production and lastly by increasing SHBG, leading to a decrease in free testosterone levels.

Sertoli cell tumors are relatively rarer and occur in younger people. They predominantly cause estrogen excess by causing a rise in aromatase activity. They are also seen as components of Peutz-Jeghers syndrome and Carney complex.

Human chorionic gonadotropin (hCG) secreting tumors can arise not only from testes, but also many other organs. Like LH, hCG stimulates Leydig cells of the testes to secrete estradiol preferentially, and it also has a role in the aromatization of other androgens to estradiol. Serum β-hCG is useful as a tumor marker in these patients.

Feminizing adrenal tumors are generally large, malignant and can occur in the young to middle aged. They often present as palpable abdominal masses and cause gynecomastia either by an absolute androgen excess, peripheral aromatization of androgen precursors or estrogen mediated LH suppression. dehydroepiandiosterone sulfate (DHEAS) levels are usually elevated and they can be visualized on ultrasound abdomen or CT abdomen, for better visualization. They are often widespread at presentation with metastases and treatment is more often than not, palliative.

Q. 10 What are the other causes of gynecomastia?

Ans. Familial aromatase excess is a disorder caused by overexpression of *CYP19A1* gene, leading to an increase in aromatization of adrenal and testicular androgens to estrogens. Affected females can present with premature thelarche and precocious puberty; affected males can present with precocious puberty and gynecomastia, though fertility is usually normal. This is one of the few disorders where aromatase inhibitors cause a marked improvement.

Hyperthyroidism can cause gynecomastia by increasing the SHBG, which causes a decline in the free testosterone levels. Treatment is by control of hyperthyroidism.

Primary hypogonadism is a common cause of gynecomastia, caused by low testosterone levels, and low testosterone leading to high LH levels, which activates aromatase, thus further skewing the testosterone to estrogen ratio. Chromosomal disorders like Klinefelter's, orchitis due to any reason including mumps orchitis, testicular trauma, torsion, surgery chemotherapy or irradiation to testes can result in gynecomastia. Klinefelter syndrome is one of the most common chromosomal disorders in male and classically presents with hypogonadism and gynecomastia (up to two-thirds of all cases of Klinefelter's). It is also associated with an increased risk of breast cancer in males. Milder variants of disorders of testicular biosynthesis like 17β-hydroxy-steroid dehydrogenase deficiency and minimal androgen insensitivity syndrome can also present with gynecomastia.

Secondary hypogonadism due to Kallmann syndrome, combined pituitary hormone deficiency, isolated hypogonadotropic hypogonadism, pituitary trauma, surgery, irradiations, infarcts, tumors or infections can also present with gynecomastia and hypogonadism.

Gynecomastia has also been reported in men with HIV. This can happen due to multiple mechanisms including liver disease, protease inhibitors and nucleoside reverse transcriptase inhibitors, hypogonadotropic hypogonadism, and refeeding mechanism after antiretroviral therapy induced weight gain.

The drugs implicated in gynecomastia are numerous and include spironolactone, antiandrogens like finasteride, cancer chemotherapeutic drugs for testicular and prostate carcinoma, ketoconazole, spironolactone, marijuana, flutamide and cimetidine which act by blocking the androgen receptors and inadvertent use of exogenous estrogens.

Q. 11 How do you evaluate a person with gynecomastia?

Ans. The crux of evaluating a person with gynecomastia lies in ruling out systemic, endocrine or neoplastic causes of gynecomastia, so that unnecessary diagnostic evaluation and treatment is avoided (Flowchart 10.1). Hence, the evaluation relies on three basic questions:

- Is this true gynecomastia?
- If this is true gynecomastia, is this physiological?
- If this is not physiological gynecomastia, what is the cause?

To answer the first question, differentiating true gynecomastia from pseudogynecomastia is best achieved by clinical examination. Most of the breast prominence is pseudogynecomastia is due to subcutaneous fat (lipomastia) and on palpation, the cord-like firm breast tissue which is palpable in true gynecomastia is never felt. Also a comparison of the subareolar mass with adjacent subcutaneous fat in the axilla helps better in differentiation.

Etiology of true gynecomastia is best achieved by taking a detailed and relevant history, physical examination and judicious use of diagnostic tests. History should include information about age of onset (for age of presentation of physiological gynecomastia, vide supra), mode of presentation (whether unilateral or bilateral, tender or nontender), history of chronic disorders (renal, hepatic, thyrotoxicosis, primary or secondary hypogonadism, medications, exposure to sources of estrogens and history of testicular or prostate carcinoma). Family history of gynecomastia—(aromatase excess) and ambiguous genitalia (androgen insensitivity) should also be recorded. Mode of onset can often give valuable clues with firm to hard breast mass, fixation to underlying structures, eccentric location and ulceration or nipple retraction, associated axillary lymph nodes and discharge (especially if bloodstained) pointing towards breast malignancy.

Physical examination should include examination for signs of all the chronic systemic diseases mentioned above, palpation for goiter and a systematic breast examination for the malignant signs elucidated above. It should also include a palpation of abdomen and scrotum and evaluation of secondary sexual characters.

Biochemical evaluation should be judicious and a basic work-up should include liver, renal and thyroid function tests, measurement of gonadotropins, testosterone and also, as and when required, estrogens, prolactin, β-hCG, α-fetoprotein and adrenal androgens like DHEAS and 17-OH progesterone (less commonly). Ultrasound of scrotum and CT abdomen are routinely not requested except when an abdominal or testicular malignancy is suspected. Mammography has a role only if breast malignancy is suspected. Men with Klinefelter syndrome need more extensive evaluation because they have a 20- to 60-fold increase in breast cancer risk compared with normal men. However, mammography is not

FLOWCHART 10.1 Management of gynecomastia

- Breast enlargement
  - Lipomastia
    - Weight loss Cosmetic surgery if required
  - Features suggestive of malignancy
    - Mammography, ultrasound, biopsy, if required and appropriate referral
  - True gynecomastia
    - Long standing painless
      - Persistent puberty gynecomastia reassure Surgery if causing cosmetic issues
    - Recent onset tender
      - Drugs
        - Stop medication
      - • Cirrhosis • Dialysis • Refeeding
        - Re-feeding mechanism
      - Pubertal
        - Watchful reassurance
      - Miscellaneous disorders
        - Evaluate for hyperthyroidism, tumors, HIV
      - Features of hypogonadism
        - Hormonal evaluation—LH, FSH, T
          - • Low T, LH, FSH • Secondary hypogonadism
          - • Low T, High LH, FSH • Primary hypogonadism
      - • No hypogonadism • Plan other hormonal work-up
        - Elevated hCG
          - Scrotal and ultrasound for hCG secreting tumor
            - If negative, imaging in other areas for hCG secreting tumor
        - Elevated estrogen
          - Look for sources of exogenous estrogens
            - If not found, imaging for estrogen-secreting tumors
        - Hormonal work-up negative
          - Idiopathic gynecomastia

Abbreviations: HIV, human immunodeficiency virus; LH, luteinizing hormone; FSH, follicle-stimulating hormone; T, testosterone; hCG, human chorionic gonadotropin

recommended as a routine, since their absolute risk of breast malignancy is still much lesser than women.

Q. 12 How do you manage a case of gynecomastia?

Ans. Management depends on the cause. If it is pseudogynecomastia, the patient needs only reassurance and advice about weight loss. If he is very self-conscious, liposuction can be advised. Physiological gynecomastia normally needs only reassurance and advice regarding weight loss, since in a lot of cases, this gynecomastia is accentuated by underlying subareolar fat. On most occasions, puberty gynecomastia regresses, but if it is persistent, cosmetic relief can be provided by surgery.

In all patients, offending medications should be stopped and underlying chronic conditions treated. If there is no response, then a trial of medical therapy can be attempted. The commonly used medications are tamoxifen, aromatase inhibitors and clomiphene. Tamoxifen is the most commonly used drug and acts by blocking the estrogen effects on breast tissue. A course of 10–20 mg/day for 3–9 months has been successfully used. If gynecomastia recurs on stopping the drug, a second course can be tried. Tamoxifen is also quite useful in gynecomastia due to antiandrogen therapy in testicular and prostate cancer. Clomiphene is on the whole, less efficacious. The aromatase inhibitors like anastrozole, letrozole and testolactone are quite effective in aromatase excess disorders, but this efficacy has not been duplicated when used for other indications.

Testosterone therapy is the treatment in all cases of gynecomastia due to absolute androgen deficiency. There might be an initial flare-up of gynecomastia due to conversion of testosterone to estrogen, but with continued therapy, gynecomastia often regresses. In men with long-standing symptomatic gynecomastia (more than 12 months), medical therapy is less likely to be effective, because the stroma is mostly fibrotic. Surgery is the treatment of choice and involves excision of the glandular tissue by a periareolar incision and fat removal, if required.

Coming back to the case, since a diagnosis of Klinefelter is made, the boy is started on testosterone therapy. He has also been placed on follow-up with the endocrinology department and has been started on a special academics programme in conjunction with the adolescent psychiatry clinics.

SUGGESTED READING

1. Bembo SA, Carlson HE. Gynecomastia: its features, and when and how to treat it. Cleve Clin J Med. 2004;71(6):511-7.
2. Braunstein GD. Clinical practice. Gynecomastia. N Engl J Med. 2007;357:1229.
3. Jacobs EC. Effect of starvation on sex hormones in the male. J Clin Endocrinol Metab. 1948;8:227-32.
4. Johnson RE, Murad MH. Gynecomastia: pathophysiology, evaluation, and management. Mayo Clin Proc. 2009;84:1010.
5. Narula HS, Carlson HE. Gynecomastia. Endocrinol Metab Clin North Am. 2007;36(2):497-519.
6. Paduch DA, Fine RG, Bolyakov A, Kiper J. New concepts in Klinefelter syndrome. Curr Opin Urol. 2008;18(6):621-7.
7. Platt SS, Schulz RZ, Kunstadter RH. Hypertrophy of the male breast associated with recovery from starvation. Bulletin of US Army Medical Department. 1947;7:403-5.
8. Sivaprakash Somasundaram, AC Ammini. Gynecomastia. Pediatric Endocrine Disorders; 2014. pp. 159-62.

CHAPTER

11

Drug-induced Thyroid Disorder

Sambit Das

CASE

Mr BK, a 55-year-old male has presented with chief complaints of generalized weakness of 2 months duration, weight loss of two months duration and intermittent palpitation for last 15 days. He is a known case of hypertension on treatment. He had an acute anterior wall myocardial infarction one year ago for which he had to undergo percutaneous transluminal coronary angioplasty. Postcoronary intervention patient developed ventricular tachycardia on three occasions (one in ICU and two times in the ward). For which, he was electroverted and was put on amiodarone (200 mg tablets three times a day since then).

Current clinical examination reveals sinus tachycardia with heart rate of 110 per minute, blood pressure is 126/80 mm Hg. He has a grade-1 soft diffuse goiter.

On evaluation, his routine hemogram with renal function and liver function tests are normal. His thyroid function test reveals serum T3 of 190 ng/dL (normal range, 80–200 ng/dL), serum T4 of 22 μg/dL (normal range 5.1–14.1 μg/dL) and serum TSH of 0.01 μIU/mL (normal range, 0.27–4.20 μIU/mL). Serum anti-TPO antibody is within normal range.

Q. 1 What is the provisional diagnosis in this case?

Ans. This is a case of thyrotoxicosis probably amiodarone induced.

Q. 2 What is amiodarone?

Ans. Amiodarone is an antiarrhythmic drug with high iodine content and high fat solubility. Structurally, the drug resembles T4 and contains 37% of iodine by weight. So each 200 mg of tablet contains 75 mg of iodine and about 6 mg of iodide is released per day. Amiodarone has a half-life of 50–60 days and hence remain for a long time in body even after its discontinuation.

Q. 3 What is the mechanism of its effect on thyroid gland?

Ans.

- It is a source of large amount of iodine to body.
- It inhibits the D1 and to some extent D2 deiodinases.
- Due to its structural similarity, it competes with T3 to bind to its receptor site.
- Direct cytotoxic effect on thyroid cell by inducing apoptosis.
- The drug and its metabolites induces autoimmune thyroid disease in susceptible individuals.

Q. 4 What is amiodarone-induced thyrotoxicosis?

Ans. Amiodarone-induced thyrotoxicosis (AIT) occurs in 2–12% of patients on chronic amiodarone treatment depending on the dietary iodine intake of the population.

Type-I AIT: This occurs in patients with preexisting thyroid abnormalities and thyrotoxicosis is believed to result from iodine-induced excessive thyroid hormone synthesis. This is an example of the Jod-Basedow phenomenon.

Type-II AIT: In patients with an apparently normal thyroid gland, thyrotoxicosis results from glandular damage with consequent release of preformed thyroid hormones into the circulation. Studies have shown amiodarone to be cytotoxic to FRTL-5 thyroid cells. On histopathology, moderate-to-severe follicular damage and disruption were demonstrated.

The finding of markedly elevated serum levels of interleukin-6 (IL-6) in type II AIT patients further supports this destructive-cum-inflammatory process. Thyrotoxicosis in type II AIT patients is usually self-limiting, which may be due to dose-dependent cytotoxic effect of the drug (Table 11.1).

Q. 5 How to diagnose amiodarone-induced thyrotoxicosis?

Ans. Clinical features of unexplained weight loss, tremor, sinus tachycardia or worsening of the underlying cardiac disorder and new onset tachyarrhythmias

TABLE 11.1 Types of amiodarone induced thyrotoxicosis

	Type I AIT	*TYPE II AIT*
Underlying thyroid abnormality	Present	Absent
Pathogenic mechanism	Jod-Basedow effect	Thyroiditis with release of hormones
Goiter	Multinodular of diffuse goiter	Occasionally small and diffuse goiter
Radioiodine uptake	Normal/raised	Low or absent
Serum IL-6	Normal	Profoundly raised
Thyroid USG	Increased volume, nodular	Normal
Color flow Doppler	High vascularity	Absent vascularity

Abbreviation: AIT, amiodarone-induced thyrotoxicosis

suggest AIT. Biochemically, there would be marked increase in serum levels of free T4 (or high total T4 and free thyroxine index), with suppressed serum TSH. Serum T3 levels in such individuals may be either marginally elevated or normal; the presentation of T4 toxicosis being one of the peculiar features of AIT.

Q. 6 How to differentiate between different types of amiodarone-induced thyrotoxicosis?

Ans. Although differentiation between the two forms of AIT may not always be feasible, this is useful to determine the most appropriate treatment. Thyroid RAIU study may be helpful in this regard, as the 24-hour uptake is usually normal-to-high in patients with type I AIT and low-to suppressed in type II AIT. The measurement of circulating IL-6 levels also appears to be a promising discriminator but this is not widely available. In a recent study, color flow Doppler sonography was found to permit rapid differentiation between the two types of AIT. In the evaluation of 27 consecutive patients, by this technique before starting antithyroid treatment, parenchymal blood flow was demonstrated in all type I AIT patients while it was absent in all type II AIT patients.

Q. 7 Describe the management of amiodarone-induced thyrotoxicosis.

Ans. Distinguishing between the two types of AIT is important because it has a major influence on subsequent management.

Type 1 AIT: Therapy for type I AIT consists of withdrawal of amiodarone (if possible) with initiation of carbimazole or methimazole.

Potassium perchlorate has been used as an adjunct in patients who are given CBZ (or MMI) to a maximum of 5 g/day. Potassium perchlorate reduces the intrathyroidal iodine stores because it decreases the entry of iodine into the thyroid and competitively inhibits thyroid iodine uptake (Basaria and Cooper, 2005). If AIT is associated with underlying Grave's disease or multinodular goiter than definitive treatment with radioablation or surgery is indicated. Before doing radioablation, iodine uptake by thyroid has to be ascertained for a better outcome.

Type-II AIT: Therapy for this type of AIT consists of possible stoppage of amiodarone with starting of oral prednisolone at 40–60 mg/day. Steroid needs to be tapered according to improvement of thyrotoxicosis. Nonspecific beta-blocker can be added for symptomatic improvement.

The patient in case 1 is started on methimazole 15 mg and is asked to follow up after 2 months. The amiodarone dose is continued as the cardiologist opined that it is not possible to reduce the dose of amiodarone at the moment.

Q. 8 How frequently do we need to monitor thyroid dysfunction in a patient on amiodarone therapy?

Ans. Amiodarone induced toxicosis may develop at the outset of its use or not until several years of its use. This serious condition can be anticipated by early recognition of progressive decline in serum thyroid-stimulating hormone (TSH). Though there is no particular guidelines for testing but it is prudent to check serum TSH every 6 months throughout the use of amiodarone therapy.

Q. 9 What is Jod-Basedow effect?

Ans. Administration of supplemental iodine to iodine deficient region may precipitate thyrotoxicosis which is otherwise known as Jod-Basedow effect. Jod is derived from a German word meaning iodine and Basedow means Graves' disease. This effect occurs in population who have partial autonomous thyroid function. There are two groups of people who develop the condition. The first group is an elderly population with multinodular goiter who have some autonomous thyroid tissue. This group lacks the thyroid autoimmune markers. The second group is a young population with mild diffuse goiter who have markers of thyroid immunity like TRAb positivity.

Q. 10 What is the amiodarone-induced hypothyroidism?

Ans. Incidence of amiodarone-induced hypothyroidism (AIH) varies widely, ranging from 6% in countries with low iodine intake to 13% in countries with a high-dietary iodine intake. The relative risk of developing AIH was found to be 13-fold higher in female patients with positive thyroid microsomal or thyroglobulin antibodies, as compared with men without thyroid antibodies. Hypothyroidism is usually an early event and it is uncommon after the first 18 months of amiodarone treatment amiodarone-induced hypothyroidism (AIH) is believed to result from the inability of the thyroid to escape from the Wolff-Chaikoff effect. Thyroid hormone biosynthesis is impaired because of the persistent block in intrathyroidal iodine organification, as evident by the positive perchlorate discharge test in patients with AIH. This may arise from an underlying thyroid abnormality, such as autoimmune thyroiditis. 40% of patients who develop hypothyroidism after amiodarone administration have positive thyroid antibodies.

Q. 11 What is the management of AIH?

Ans. Management consists of discontinuation of amiodarone (if possible) with starting of levothyroxine. Monitoring should be done every 6 weeks and serum T4 is to kept at upper normal range.

Q. 12 What is dronedarone?

Ans. Dronedarone is a noniodinated benzofuran derivative of amiodarone in which the iodine moieties, observed with amiodarone, are substituted with a methyosulfonamide group. Hence, dronedarone is less lipophilic than amiodarone, with a much shorter half-life (24 hours) than amiodarone.

Q. 13 What other drugs can cause thyroid dysfunction?

Ans. See Boxes 11.1 and 11.2.

Q. 14 What is the mechanism of lithium-induced hypothyroidism?

Ans. Lithium increases intrathyroidal iodine content and inhibits the uncoupling of residues to form iodothyronines (thyroxine [T4] and triiodothyronine [T3]). It also inhibits the release of T3 and T4. It also decreases peripheral deiodination of tetraiodothyronine (T4) or thyroxine by decreasing the activity of type I 5' deiodinase enzyme.

BOX 11.1 Drugs and agents causing hypothyroidism

- Drugs which inhibit release of thyroid hormones or synthesis—lithium, amiodarone and other iodine containing drugs, thioamides, perchlorate, radiographic agents, potassium Iodide solution, aminoglutethimide, thalidomide
- All the agents containing iodine listed in Box 11.2 can also cause hypothyroidism
- Peripheral deiodination of tetraiodothyronine (T4) or thyroxine by decreasing the activity of type I 5′ deiodinase enzyme—lithium
- Decrease absorption of T4-proton pump inhibitors, cholestyramine, colestipol, colesevelam, calcium carbonate, sucralfate, ferrous sulfate, raloxifene, aluminum hydroxide
- Immune dysregulation-interleukin 2, interferon-alpha, ipilimumab, alemtuzumab, pembrolizumab
- Suppression of TSH—dopamine
- Destructive thyroiditis—sunitinib
- Increase type 3 deiodination—sorafenib
- Increase clearance of T4 NDs suppression of TSH-Bexarotene
- Iodine
- Lithium
- Tyrosine kinase inhibitors

BOX 11.2 Drugs and agents causing hyperthyroidism

- Stimulation of release of thyroid hormone or synthesis of thyroid hormone-amiodarone
- Iodine containing agents such as radiographic agents, e.g. diatrizoate, iopanoic acid, ipodate, iothalamate, metrizamide, diatrozide, topical iodine preparation-like tincture iodine, povidone iodine, Iodoform gauge
- Solutions such as saturated solution of potassium iodide (SSKI), Lugols iodine, Iodinated glycerol; expectorants, vitamins-containing iodine, iodochlorohydroxyquinoline, di-iodohydroxyquinoline, potassium iodide, benziodarone, isopropamide iodide
- Food components such as Kelp, kombu and other algae
- Food colors such as erythrosine
- Iodine containing food such as hamburger thyroiditis
- Immune dysregulation-interleukin 2, interferon-alpha, ipilimumab, alemtuzumab, pembrolizumab

Q. 15 In what all ways lithium can affect the thyroid gland?

Ans. Lithium can cause goiter, hypothyroidism, rarely hyperthyroidism/ thyrotoxicosis and possibly has some relationship with thyroid autoimmunity and development of hyperthyroidism. Goiter and hypothyroidism are more common with the use of lithium which can occur in 40–50% and 20–30% patients, respectively.

Q. 16 Can lithium cause autoimmunity?

Ans. It has been shown in studies that patients who are on lithium treatment may have more prevalence of antibodies. The mechanism is probably augmentation of the activity of B lymphocytes and reduction of the ratio of circulating suppressor to cytotoxic T-cells.

Q. 17 Can lithium cause hyperthyroidism/thyrotoxicosis?

Ans. The frequency of hyperthyroidism in patients treated with lithium has been found to be two to three times higher than in the general population.

Q. 18 What is the probable mechanism of hyperthyroidism/thyrotoxicosis induced by lithium?

Ans. Lithium-induced hyperthyroidism is mainly characterized by a transient and painless thyroiditis. Some studies have also shown that lithium is associated with granulomatous thyroiditis, lymphocytic thyroiditis or nonspecific thyroiditis. Lithium increases the B-cell activity, and decreases the ratio of cytotoxic to suppressor T-cells and thus has been found to trigger autoimmunity which can precipitate hyperthyroidism also.

Q. 19 What is the cause of goiter?

Ans. The initial inhibition of thyroid hormone synthesis and release by lithium results into increased TSH concentrations leading to thyroid enlargement. Other mechanisms which have been proposed to explain thyrocyte proliferation among patients. Lithium therapy include activation of the pro-proliferative tyrosine kinase and Wnt/β-catenin signaling pathways.

Q. 20 What should be done when starting lithium treatment?

Ans. A thyroid function tests and titer of anti-TPO antibodies should be done before starting lithium treatment.

Patients who are euthyroid at the start of treatment should be re-evaluated every 6–12 months for several years.

SUGGESTED READING

1. Barvalia U, Amlani B, Pathak R. Amiodarone-induced thyrotoxic thyroiditis: adiagnostic and therapeutic challenge. Case Rep Med. 2014;2014:231651. doi:10.1155/2014/231651. Epub, 2014.
2. Bogazzi F, Tomisti L, Bartalena L, Aghini-Lombardi F, Martino E. Amiodarone and the thyroid: a 2012 update. J Endocrinol Invest. 2012;35(3):340-8. doi:10.3275/8298. Epub 2012. Review.
3. Danzi S, Klein I. Amiodarone-induced thyroid dysfunction. J Intensive Care Med. 2015;30(4):179-85. doi: 10.1177/0885066613503278. Epub 2013.
4. Kibirige D, Luzinda K, Ssekitoleko R. Spectrum of lithium induced thyroid abnormalities: a current perspective. Thyroid Res. 2013;6(1):3. doi:10.1186/1756-6614-6-3.
5. Kopp P. Thyrotoxicosis of other Etiologies. 2010 Dec 1. In: De Groot LJ, Beck-Peccoz P, Chrousos G, Dungan K, Grossman A, Hershman JM, Koch C, McLachlan R, New M, Rebar R, Singer F, Vinik A, Weickert MO (Eds). Endotext [Internet]. South Dartmouth (MA): MDText.com, Inc.; 2000-. Available from *http://www.ncbi.nlm.nih.gov/books/NBK285562/PubMed PMID: 25905417.*
6. Thaker VV, Leung AM, Braverman LE, Brown RS, Levine B. Iodine-induced hypothyroidism in full-term infants with congenital heart disease: more common than currently appreciated? J Clin Endocrinol Metab. 2014;99(10):3521-6. doi: 10.1210/jc.2014-1956. Epub 2014.

CHAPTER

12

Approach to Male Infertility

Sunil Kota, V Sri Nagesh, Manzer AS, Altamash Shaikh

CASE

A 33-year-old man is referred for evaluation of male infertility. He and his 29 years old wife have been trying to conceive for last 2 years. She is gravida (G0), para (P0) with complete medical evaluation revealing regular ovulatory cycles and normal reproductive anatomy with no history of reproductive tract disorders, pelvic infection or surgery. The couple has had unprotected vaginal intercourse at least 2–3 times a week, having undergone a normal puberty and well previously, he complains of poor libido and poor erection with decreased volume of ejaculate for past 1 year. He shaves once a week. There is no past history of any chronic ailments or any reproductive disorders, and has taken no medications or any illicit drugs. He has no family history of hypogonadism, cleft palate or infertility; he has 2 brothers who have fathered children. He works as a software professional with no habitual smoking or drinking. He has never fathered a child. He is well virilized with normal male voice and normal upper/lower segment ratio. His body mass index (BMI) is 33.5 kg/m^2 with bilateral nontender gynecomastia; a normal genitourinary examination with normally descended testes that are 12 mL bilaterally and easily palpable vasa deferentia. His laboratory tests (performed at 8.00 am) reveal total testosterone 220 ng/dL (N: 300–1000 ng/dL), luteinizing hormone (LH)-2 mIU/mL, follicle stimulating hormone (FSH)-6 mIU/mL. Hematogram, urine analysis, hepatic and renal profiles, serum prolactin, thyroid profile and iron studies are normal. Repeat hormonal analysis reveal similar results. The seminal fluid analysis yields no sperms with volume of 2.45 mL, normal pH (≥7.2) and fructose. Repeat semen analysis shows similar results. Sella imaging reveals no hypothalamic/pituitary abnormality.

Q. 1 What is the definition of infertility and fecundability?

Ans. Infertility is a unique medical condition involving a couple, rather than a single individual. It is defined as failure of a couple to conceive after 12 months of regular intercourse without use of contraception in women less than 35 years of age; and after six months of regular intercourse without use of contraception in women 35 years and older. The frequency of sexual intercourse should be 2–3 times weekly in order to optimize the likelihood of conception.

Fecundability is the probability of achieving a pregnancy in one menstrual cycle. It is a more accurate descriptor because it recognizes varying degrees of infertility.

Q. 2 What are the normal trends of fertility?

Ans. About 85% of women conceive within 12 months. Fecundability is 0.25 in the first three months, and then decreases to 0.15 during the next nine months. Up to 50% of young, healthy couples that fail to conceive in the first 12 months will conceive in the following 12 months.

In general, women who are under age 30, who have a less than two-year history of infertility, who have had a previous pregnancy, and who do not have tubal disease, anovulation, partners with male factor infertility, or endometriosis, have the best prognosis for treatment-independent conception.

Q. 3 What is the indication and timing of infertility evaluation?

Ans.

- Initiate evaluation after 12 months of unprotected and frequent intercourse:
  - Women under age 35 years without risk factors for infertility.
- Initiate evaluation after six months of unprotected and frequent intercourse:
  - Women age 35–40 years.
- Initiate evaluation upon presentation despite less than six months of unprotected and frequent intercourse:
  - Women over age 40 years.
  - Women with oligomenorrhea/amenorrhea.
  - Women with a history of chemotherapy, radiation therapy, or advanced stage endometriosis.
  - Women with known or suspected uterine/tubal disease.
  - Women whose male partner has a history of groin or testicular surgery, adult mumps, impotence or other sexual dysfunction, chemotherapy and/or radiation, or a history of subfertility with another partner.

Q. 4 What is the gender distribution with regards to etiology of infertility?

Ans. According to a World Health Organization (WHO) multicenter health study, 20% of cases are attributed to male factors, 38% are attributed to female factors, 27% have causal factors identified in both partners, and 15% could not be satisfactorily attributed to either partner.

Q. 5 What are the causes of male infertility?

Ans. Causes of male infertility are mentioned in Box 12.1.

- Hypothalamic pituitary disease (secondary hypogonadism)—1–2%
- Testicular disease (primary testicular defects including Y chromosome microdeletions)—30–40%
- Post-testicular defects (disorders of sperm transport)—10–20%
- Idiopathic—40–50%

BOX 12.1 Causes of male infertility

- *Hypothalamic-pituitary disorders (GnRH; LH and FSH deficiency)*
  - Congenital disorders
    - Congenital GnRH deficiency (Kallmann syndrome)
    - Hemochromatosis
    - Multiorgan genetic disorders (Prader-Willi syndrome, Laurence-Moon-Biedl syndrome, familial cerebellar ataxia)
  - Acquired disorders
    - Pituitary and hypothalamic tumors (macroadenoma, craniopharyngioma)
    - Infiltrative disorders (sarcoidosis, histiocytosis, tuberculosis, fungal infections)
    - Trauma, postsurgery, postirradiation
    - Vascular (infarction, aneurysm)
    - Hormonal (hyperprolactinemia, thyroid dysfunction, androgen/estrogen excess, cortisol excess)
    - Drugs (opioids and psychotropic drugs, GnRH agonists or antagonists)
    - Systemic disorders
    - Chronic illnesses
    - Nutritional deficiencies
    - Obesity
- *Primary gonadal disorders*
  - Congenital disorders
    - Klinefelter's syndrome (XXY) and its variants (XXY/XY; XXXY)
    - Cryptorchidism
    - Myotonic dystrophy
    - Functional prepubertal castrate syndrome (congenital anorchia)
    - Varicocele
    - Androgen insensitivity syndromes
    - 5-alpha-reductase deficiency
    - Y chromosome deletions
  - Acquired disorders
    - Viral orchitis (mumps, echovirus, arbovirus)
    - Granulomatous orchitis (leprosy, tuberculosis)
    - Epididymo-orchitis (gonorrhea, chlamydia)
    - Drugs (e.g. alkylating agents, alcohol, marijuana, antiandrogens, ketoconazole, spironolactone, histamine 2 receptor antagonists)
    - Ionizing radiation
    - Environmental toxins (e.g. dibromochloropropane, carbon disulfide, cadmium, lead, mercury, environmental estrogens and phytoestrogens)
    - Hyperthermia
    - Immunologic disorders, including polyglandular autoimmune disease
    - Trauma
    - Torsion
    - Castration
    - Systemic illness (e.g. renal failure, hepatic cirrhosis, cancer, sickle cell disease, amyloidosis, vasculitis, celiac disease)
- *Disorders of sperm transport*
  - Epididymal dysfunction (drugs, infection)
  - Abnormalities of the vas deferens (congenital absence, Young's syndrome, infection, vasectomy)
  - Ejaculatory dysfunction (spinal cord disease, autonomic dysfunction, premature ejaculation, retrograde ejaculation)
- *Unexplained male factor infertility*

Q. 6 What are the components of the evaluation of an infertile man?

Ans.

- History
- Physical examination
- Semen analyses
- Genetic tests
- Endocrine testing.

Q. 7 What are the relevant points to be covered in evaluation of clinical history?

Ans.

- Developmental history, including testicular descent, pubertal development, loss of body hair, or decrease in shaving frequency.
- Chronic medical illness.
- Symptoms of thyroid disease, corticosteroid excess: Hypothalamicopituitary masses (e.g. headaches and visual changes), or acromegaly. In patients with long-standing diabetes mellitus and neurological disorders, gastrointestinal symptoms such as postprandial fullness or vomiting, chronic diarrhea or constipation might indicate dysautonomia and greater risk of ejaculatory dysfunction. Postcoital micturition that is cloudy might indicate retrograde ejaculation.
- Infections, such as mumps orchitis, sinopulmonary symptoms, sexually transmitted infections, and genitourinary tract infections including prostatitis.
- Surgical procedures involving the inguinal and scrotal areas such as vasectomy, orchiectomy, and herniorrhaphy.
- Drugs and environmental exposures, including alcohol, radiation therapy, anabolic steroids, cytotoxic chemotherapy, drugs that cause hyperprolactinemia, and exposure to toxic chemicals (e.g. pesticides, hormonal disrupters).
- Sexual history, including libido, morning erections, frequency of intercourse, sexual dysfunction (erectile dysfunction, anorgasmia), pain or abnormal curvature with erections, loss of body hairs with decreased frequency of shaving, small or shrinking testes with enlargement of breasts and previous fertility assessments of the man and his partner.
- School performance, to determine if he has a history of learning disabilities suggestive of Klinefelter's syndrome.

Q. 8 What are various components of physical examination in an infertile male?

Ans. The physical examination should include a general medical examination with a focus on finding evidence of androgen deficiency. The clinical manifestations of androgen deficiency depend upon the age of onset. Androgen deficiency during early gestation presents as ambiguous genitalia; in late gestation as micropenis; in childhood as delayed pubertal development; and in adulthood as decreased sexual function, infertility, and eventually, loss of secondary sex characteristics. The examination of the man should include the following components:

General appearance—eunuchoidal proportions (upper/lower body ratio <1 with an arm span 5 cm >standing height) suggest androgen deficiency antedating puberty. On the other hand, increased body fat and decreased muscle mass suggest current androgen deficiency.

Skin—loss of pubic, axillary, and facial hair, decreased oiliness of the skin, and fine facial wrinkling suggest long-standing androgen deficiency.

External genitalia—several abnormalities that can affect fertility can be recognized by examination of the external genitalia:

- The penis should be examined for any hypospadias and fibrosis.
- Incomplete sexual development can be recognized by examining the phallus and testes and finding a Tanner stage other than 5.
- Diseases that affect sperm maturation and transport can be detected by examination of the scrotum for absence of the vas, epididymal thickening, varicocele, and hernia. The presence of a varicocele should be confirmed with the man in recumbent and standing positions and performing a Valsalva maneuver; varicoceles should shrink significantly in the recumbent position. The testes should be carefully palpated for masses; testicular cancer is more prevalent in infertile men.
- Decreased volume of the seminiferous tubules can be detected by measuring testicular size by Prader orchidometer. In an adult man, testicular volume below 15 mL and testicular length below 3.6 cm are considered small. In infertile men with testes <15 cc, there generally is a direct correlation between testicular volume and successful medical treatment of fertility. A testicular volume >6 cc generally portends a better response to treatment.
- Breasts—gynecomastia suggests a decreased androgen to estrogen ratio.

Q. 9 What are the parameters of standard semen analysis?

Ans. The semen sample should be collected after two to seven days of sexual abstinence, preferably at the doctor's office by masturbation. If this is not possible, then the samples can be collected with condoms without chemical additives and delivered to the laboratory within an hour of collection.

The standard semen analysis consists of the following:

- Measurement of semen volume and pH
- Microscopy for debris and agglutination
- Assessment of sperm concentration, motility, and morphology
- Sperm leukocyte count
- Search for immature germ cells.

Q. 10. What are the lower reference limits for various parameters?

Ans. The WHO, in 2010 has published revised lower reference limits for semen analyses, which is depicted in Box 12.2.

Semen volume: Aspermia or complete absence of ejaculation can be due to congenital absence of vas deferens or ejaculatory duct obstruction. Low semen volume with normal sperm concentration is most likely due to semen collection problems (loss of a portion of the ejaculate) and partial retrograde

BOX 12.2 WHO prescribed lower reference limits for semen analysis

- Volume—1.5 mL
- Sperm concentration—15 million spermatozoa/mL
- Total sperm number—39 million spermatozoa per ejaculate
- Morphology—4% normal forms (95% CI 3–4), using "strict" Tygerberg method
- Vitality—58% live
- Progressive motility—32%
- Total (progressive + nonprogressive motility)—40%

ejaculation. Androgen deficiency is also associated with low semen volume and low sperm concentration. The patient should be asked to return for a carefully collected repeat semen sample after emptying the bladder; post ejaculation urine can be collected to assess whether there is retrograde ejaculation.

Sperm concentration: Lack of sperm in the ejaculate does not indicate the absence of testicular sperm production; these patients should be evaluated for retrograde ejaculation, congenital absence of the vas deferens, and other causes of obstructive azoospermia.

Sperm morphology: The criteria for normal morphology include shape, length, width, width ratio, area occupied by the acrosome, and neck and tail defects. These criteria are called "strict" criteria and have good predictive value in terms of fertilization in vitro and pregnancy rates after *in vitro* fertilization (IVF).

Leukocytes: Polymorphonuclear leukocytes, are frequently present in the seminal fluid. Assessment of white blood cells is usually performed by using the peroxidase stain. The peroxidase positive cells are counted using the hemocytometer. Presence of increased white blood cells in the ejaculate may be a marker of genital infection/inflammation and may be associated with poor semen quality because of the release of reactive oxygen species from the leukocytes. The suggested cut-off for the diagnosis of a possible infection is one million leukocytes/mL of ejaculate.

Q. 11 What are the other specialized semen tests?

Ans.

- Sperm autoantibodies
- Semen biochemistry (semen fructose)
- Semen culture
- Sperm-cervical mucus interaction tests
- Sperm function tests
  - Computer-aided sperm analysis
  - Acrosome reaction
  - Zona free hamster oocyte penetration test
  - Human zona pellucida binding test
  - Sperm reactive oxygen species generation
- Sperm chromatin/DNA assays.

Q. 12 How to evaluate obstructive azoospermia?

Ans. If a patient has normal testicular volumes, normal serum follicle-stimulating hormone (FSH), and luteinizing hormone (LH) and testosterone and azoospermia, the likely diagnosis is obstructive azoospermia (Flowchart 12.1). The bilateral congenital absence of the vas can be detected on physical examination along with low seminal fluid volume and acidic pH.

FLOWCHART 12.1 Approach to male infertility

Male infertility

History, physical examination, semen analysis

Reduced sperm count, often with abnormal morphology and <50% motility

Normal sperm count with abnormal morphology or decreased motility

Normal, with no abnormality in female

Repeat semen analysis

Normal, with no abnormality in female

Abnormal

Specialized tests of sperm function

Measure serum T, FSH, LH

↓ T
↑ FSH
↑ LH

Normal T
↑ FSH
Normal LH

Normal T
Normal FSH
Normal LH

↓ T
↓ FSH
↓ LH

↑ T
Normal FSH
↑ LH

Primary panhypogonadism

Germinal epithelium failure

Hypogonadotropic hypogonadism

Partial androgen resistance

Seek other causes

Azoo- or severe oligozoospermia: Karyotype and Y chromosome microdeletions

Retrieve ejaculate or testicular sperm for ICSI

It is confirmed by a low/absent fructose level in the semen. Ejaculatory duct obstruction presents with normal semen fructose, normal sized testes. It is diagnosed by a transrectal ultrasound showing dilated seminal vesicles, fine needle aspiration or open biopsy of the testis should be considered to demonstrate the presence of normal testicular histology. Patients with obstructive azoospermia should be referred to a urologist specialized in infertility for further evaluation and treatment. IVF and ICSI serve as the best options of treatment.

Q. 13 What are the various endocrine tests for evaluation of an infertile male?

Ans. Serum testosterone, luteinizing hormone (LH), and follicle-stimulating hormone (FSH), prolactin, thyroid function test.

Serum testosterone: Measurement of a morning serum total testosterone is usually sufficient. In men with borderline values, the measurement should be repeated and measurement of serum free testosterone may be helpful.

Serum LH and FSH: When the serum testosterone concentration is low, high serum FSH and LH concentrations indicate primary hypogonadism and values that are low or normal indicate secondary hypogonadism. In cases of secondary hypogonadism, other pituitary hormones are also to be evaluated.

Men with low sperm counts and low serum LH concentrations (+ low Sex hormone binding globulin) who are well-androgenized (acne, increased muscularity) with soft testes should be suspected of exogenous anabolic or androgenic steroid abuse. Approach to male infertility is mentioned in Flowchart 12.1.

Q. 14 When to order for a scrotal ultrasound?

Ans. If there is a scrotal abnormality on examination, if there is a testicular mass suspected on examination, or if the scrotal examination is difficult (e.g. retracted testes) or those at risk for testicular cancer, e.g. cryptorchidism or past history of testicular cancer.

Q. 15. What are the various forms of treatment for male infertility?

Ans.

- Specific treatment is available only for infertility due to hypogonadotropic hypogonadism
  - *Hyperprolactinemia:* Discontinuation of causal medication, treatment with dopamine agonist, such as cabergoline or bromocriptine. Normal spermatogenesis takes three months. As a result, restoration of a normal sperm count usually does not occur for at least three and sometimes six months or more after the serum prolactin and testosterone concentrations have returned to normal.
  - *Other causes:* Gonadotropin therapy—treatment is initiated with human chorionic gonadotropin (hCG), 1500–2000 IU 2–3 times per week subcutaneously or intramuscularly for at least six months. hCG has the biologic activity of luteinizing hormone. The hCG dose should be adjusted upward according to symptoms of hypogonadism, serum testosterone concentrations, and semen parameters. Some patients

with acquired hypogonadotropic states (pretreatment testes ≥ 8 cc) can be stimulated with hCG alone to produce sufficient sperm. If after six to nine months the patient remains azoospermic or severely oligospermic (<10 million/mL), then human menopausal gonadotropin (hMG) or recombinant follicle-stimulating hormone (FSH) at dosage of 150 IU thrice a week should be added. The dosage of FSH may be doubled if conception has not occurred and sperm concentrations remain < 20 million/mL within 6 months of initiation of combination therapy with hCG. On average, conception occurs after 2–3 years of gonadotropin therapy and occurs when sperm concentrations are between 5 and 20 million/mL, men with postpubertal gonadotropin deficiency might respond to hCG monotherapy, but men with prepubertal onset of gonadotropin deficiency virtually always benefit from combination hCG plus FSH therapy.

An FSH level greater than 8 IU/L should raise the suspicion of primary spermatogenic failure; gonadotropin therapy is unlikely to improve fertility. In general, gonadotropin therapy is not useful for men with idiopathic infertility.

Pulsatile gonadotropin-releasing hormone (GnRH) therapy—only men who have hypogonadotropic hypogonadism due to hypothalamic disease can be treated with GnRH. GnRH has to be delivered in pulses using a portable pump with an attached catheter and needle for many months or years; most patients find it inconvenient to use GnRH therapy for so long.

- Treatment of uncertain efficacy:

Etiology	*General aspects of treatment*
Infections	Antibiotics least a 10-day course of antibiotics such as erythromycin or trimethoprim-sulfamethoxazole or a quinolone
Sperm autoimmunity	High-dose glucocorticoids (prednisone (from 40 to 80 mg/day) for up to six months); assisted reproductive techniques—intracytoplasmic sperm injection (ICSI)
Sexual dysfunction	Appropriate therapy
Retrograde ejaculation	Alpha agonist therapy. Intrauterine insemination (IUI) with washed spermatozoa or assisted reproductive techniques
Varicocele	High ligation or embolization of spermatic veins
Obstructive azoospermia	Microsurgical end-to-end anastomoses (epididymal ducts to epididymal ducts or to vas); microsurgical epididymal sperm aspiration and *in vitro* fertilization/ICSI

- *Empirical therapy:* Antiestrogens (Clomiphene citrate), aromatase inhibitors (letrozole, anastrozole), vitamin E, pentoxifylline, kallikrein, zinc, arginine, etc.
- *Assisted reproductive techniques:* In infertile couples, 40–45% of ART procedures (including ICSI) result in pregnancy.

- *Intrauterine insemination:* The intrauterine insemination (IUI) procedure consists of washing an ejaculated semen specimen to remove prostaglandins, concentrating the sperm in a small volume of culture media, and injecting the sperm suspension directly into the upper uterine cavity using a small catheter threaded through the cervix. The insemination is timed to take place just prior to ovulation, typically using home urine luteinizing hormone (LH) measurement.
- *In vitro* fertilization (IVF) is employed using the ejaculated sperm from a man with moderate oligospermia.
- Intracytoplasmic sperm injection (ICSI) has revolutionized the treatment and improved the prognosis for fertility of men with very severe oligospermia, asthenospermia (low sperm motility), teratospermia (a higher rate of abnormal sperm morphology), and even azoospermia. This technique involves the direct injection of a single spermatozoon into the cytoplasm of a human oocyte, usually obtained from follicles produced under controlled ovarian hyperstimulation.

  Approximately 10–18% of infertile men, previously classified as having idiopathic oligozoospermia, have microdeletions of the Y chromosome. Complete deletions of the AZFa or AFZb regions lead to azoospermia and Sertoli cell only syndrome. A substantial number of men with known causes of infertility also have Y chromosome microdeletions, but such deletions are rare in men with sperm concentrations over 5 million/mL. Yq microdeletions are the most common identifiable genetic cause of spermatogenic failure in around 4% of oligozoospermic men. AZFc deletion accounts for approximately 60% of Y microdeletions. These Y chromosome deletions may be transmitted from father to son by ICSI. In addition, low-level sex chromosome mosaicism has been reported in infertile couples. Therefore, genetic counseling and chromosome and other molecular genetic tests are undertaken before ICSI is undertaken. Routine karyotyping is recommended for infertile men with spermatogenic failure and a sperm concentration less than 10 million/mL and all subfertile men with hypergonadotropic hypogonadism.

  Testing for Y chromosome microdeletions should also be considered for all men with idiopathic spermatogenic deficiency and pretreatment sperm concentrations < 5 million/mL; some experts use a threshold of < 10 million/mL. All men with congenital bilateral or unilateral absence of a vas deferens should be screened for gene mutations associated with cystic fibrosis.
- Retrieval of sperm from the testis—new surgical techniques have been introduced to retrieve spermatozoa from patients with nonobstructive azoospermia. A technique called microdissection of the testis to extract sperm (TESE) from the seminiferous tubules has been successful in obtaining sperm in over 50% of patients with nonobstructive azoospermia, including patients with Klinefelter syndrome.

- *Causes of male factor infertility for which medical treatment is not available*
  - Klinefelter syndrome or variants
  - Y chromosome microdeletions (azoospermia and hyalinized tubules)
  - Sertoli cell only syndrome
  - Germ cell arrest at primary spermatocyte or earlier stage
  - *Other:* Idiopathic, cryptorchidism, postirradiation or postchemotherapy (azoospermia associated with hyalinized tubules or Sertoli cells only)

Possible treatment options include donor sperm, possible germ cell transplantation or cultured testicular stem cells.

Q. 16 Treatment options for the patient discussed.

Ans. This patient has a presentation consistent with adult onset idiopathic hypogonadotropic hypogonadism. The patient is advised to quit smoking and refrain from excessive drinking. He is advised to lose 5–10% of body weight via lifestyle changes. His symptoms of low libido and his low serum T and inappropriately normal gonadotropin levels suggest hypogonadotropism. His physical examination, normal seminal fluid volume, pH and fructose levels make obstruction unlikely. By history and evaluation, the wife is likely to be ovulatory and fertile. The patient would be offered gonadotropin therapy. It is reasonable to offer hCG therapy followed by rhFSH therapy if necessary. His testicular volumes are >6 cc; his sperm concentrations might rapidly increase with hCG therapy alone. Recombinant FSH would be added after 6 months of hCG if conception has not occurred and sperm concentration remains <10 million/mL. I would discuss the option of referral for ART without gonadotropin therapy now, but a short course of gonadotropin therapy might obviate the need for ART or improve the success rate of ART. Because his wife is 29 years old and close to entering the typical time for declining fertility, he should not be treated with gonadotropin therapy for more than 12–15 months before considering ART. If he has persistent absence of spermatogenesis despite gonadotropin therapy, the diagnosis of adult onset idiopathic hypogonadotropic hypogonadism must be reconsidered. He then must be treated as a man with idiopathic spermatogenic failure, and he should be provided genetic counseling before offering genetic testing or initiating ART.

KEY POINTS

- Infertility is defined as failure of a couple to conceive after 12 months of regular intercourse without use of contraception. The frequency of sexual intercourse should be 2–3 times weekly
- Twenty percent of cases are attributed to male factors, 38% are attributed to female factors, 27% have causal factors identified in both partners, and 15% could not be satisfactorily attributed to either partner
- Most common cause of male infertility is idiopathic followed by testicular disease, post-testicular defects and hypothalamic pituitary disease

- WHO prescribed lower reference limits for semen analyses include volume—1.5 mL, sperm concentration—15 million/mL, total sperm number—39 million per ejaculate, morphology—4% normal forms, vitality—58% live, progressive motility—32% and total (progressive + nonprogressive motility)-40%
- Basic endocrine evaluation includes serum testosterone, luteinizing hormone (LH), and follicle-stimulating hormone (FSH), prolactin, thyroid function test
- Specific treatment is available only for infertility due to hypogonadotropic hypogonadism like dopamine receptor agonists for hyperprolactinemia and gonadotropin therapy
- In infertile couples, 40–45% of ART procedures (including ICSI) result in pregnancy.

SUGGESTED READING

1. Gnoth C, Godehardt E, Frank-Herrmann P, Friol K, Tigges J, Freundl G. Definition and prevalence of subfertility and infertility. Hum Reprod. 2005;20:1144-7.
2. Jungwirth A, Giwercman A, Tournaye H, et al. 2012 European Association of Urology Guidelines on Male Infertility: the 2012 update. Eur Urol. 2012;62:324-32.
3. Male Infertility Best Practice Policy Committee of the American Urological Association; Practice Committee of the American Society for Reproductive Medicine. Report on optimal evaluation of the infertile male. Fertil Steril. 2006;86(5 Suppl 1):S202-S9.
4. Rowland D, McMahon CG, Abdo C, et al. Disorders of orgasm and ejaculation in men. J Sex Med. 2010;7:1668-86.

CHAPTER

13

Adrenal Incidentaloma

BS Narendra, Chitra S

CASE 1

A 22-year-old female comes with an incidentally detected mass in the right adrenal gland of 2 cm size detected during a CT scan done for abdominal pain. She has no hypertension, no cushingoid features and no virilization. She has no family history of multiple endocrine neoplasia. She has no history of renal calculi. The cause of abdominal pain is finally diagnosed as abdominal migraine. How will you evaluate this case of adrenal incidentaloma?

An adrenal "incidentaloma" is an adrenal mass, generally 1 cm or more in diameter that is discovered 'incidentally' during a radiologic examination performed for indications other than an evaluation for adrenal disease. The definition of incidentaloma excludes patients undergoing imaging procedures as part of staging and work-up for cancer and patients with symptomatic adrenal disease not elicited due to oversight.

Adrenal incidentaloma is not a single entity; rather it is an 'umbrella' definition comprising a spectrum of different pathological entities that share the same path of discovery. The widespread use of computed tomography (CT), diagnostic ultrasound, and magnetic resonance imaging (MRI) has resulted in the frequent incidental discovery of asymptomatic adrenal masses.

The optimal diagnostic approach to a patient who has an adrenal incidentaloma is by taking a careful history and performing a physical examination, focusing on the signs and symptoms suggestive of adrenal hyperfunction or malignant disease followed by hormonal testing, when indicated. The two important questions to be answered at the end of evaluation are:

- Does the patient have a lesion suggestive of malignancy?
- Is the lesion hormonally active?
- Do you want any further information from the CT scan done?

Q. 1 What are the causes of an incidental adrenal mass in the population?

Ans. Adrenal mass could either be benign or malignant lesions. There is consistent evidence that most adrenal incidentalomas are benign, adrenal adenomas that account for 80% of all tumors.

- 80%—nonfunctioning adenoma
- 5%—subclinical Cushing syndrome
- 5%—pheochromocytoma
- 1%—aldosteronoma
- <5%—adrenocortical carcinoma (ACC)
- 2.5%—metastatic lesion
- Remaining incidentalomas were ganglioneuromas, myelolipomas, or benign cysts.

Q. 2 What is the frequency of an incidental adrenal mass in the population?

Ans. In radiological studies, the frequency of adrenal incidentalomas was estimated at 4% in middle age and increases up to more than 10% in the elderly, peaking around the fifth and seventh decade. The frequency of adrenal incidentalomas is very low in childhood and adolescence. The prevalence of adrenal incidentalomas (AIs) has been reported as high as 8% in autopsy series and 4% in radiologic series. As improved imaging techniques become available and the frequency of abdominal imaging increases, the radiologic prevalence is expected to continue escalating and concerning is the evidence supporting increased prevalence with age.

Q. 3 How do characteristic features on radiological imaging help in the evaluation of adrenal incidentaloma?

Ans. Advances in modern imaging have made it a powerful ally in delineating benign from malignant processes in AIs.

Certain characteristic features on imaging will help to distinguish among adrenal adenoma, adrenal carcinoma, pheochromocytoma, and metastatic lesions. It is important to emphasize that imaging cannot reliably distinguish between functioning and nonfunctioning adrenal adenomas as shown in Table 13.1.

- The size of the mass and its appearance on imaging are the two major predictors of malignant disease.
- *Size of adrenal mass:* Diameter greater than 4 cm was shown to have 90% sensitivity for the detection of adrenocortical carcinoma but nondiagnostic of malignancy as only 24% of lesions greater than 4 cm in diameter were malignant. Also a size less than 4 cm does not rule out malignancy.
- *Imaging phenotype:* CT features used to distinguish adenomas from nonadenomas are the lipid content of the adrenal mass and rapidity of the washout of contrast medium.
  - The intracytoplasmic fat in adenomas results in low attenuation on unenhanced CT, nonadenomas have higher attenuation on unenhanced CT. Lesions that have an attenuation value below 10 HU on noncontrast CT scan are adenomas. That being said, it is important to remember that the lipid poor variants of adenomas will have higher attenuation on unenhanced CT.
  - On contrast study, benign adrenal lesions will commonly enhance up to 80–90 HU and washout more than 50% on the delayed scan, whereas lesions such as metastatic tumors, carcinomas, or pheochromocytomas

TABLE 13.1 Characteristics of adrenal incidentalomas on imaging

Variable	*Adrenocortical adenoma*	*Adrenocortical carcinoma*	*Pheochromocytoma*	*Metastasis*
Size	Small, usually ≤3 cm in diameter	Large, usually >4 cm in diameter	Large, usually >3 cm in diameter	Variable, frequently <3
Shape	Round or oval, with smooth margins	Irregular, with unclear margins	Round or oval, with clear margins	Oval or irregular, with unclear margins
Texture	Homogeneous	Heterogeneous, with mixed densities	Heterogeneous, with cystic areas	Heterogeneous, with mixed densities
Laterality	Usually solitary and unilateral	Usually solitary, unilateral	Usually solitary, unilateral	Often bilateral
Attenuation (density) on unenhanced CT	≤10 Hounsfield units	>10 Hounsfield units (usually >25)	>10 Hounsfield units (usually >25)	>10 Hounsfield units (usually >25)
Vascularity on contrast-enhanced CT	Not highly vascular	Usually vascular	Usually vascular	Usually vascular
Rapidity of washout of contrast medium	≥50% at 10 minutes	<50% at 10 minutes	<50% at 10 minutes	<50% at 10 minutes
Appearance on MRI	Isointense in relation to liver on T2-weighted image	Hyperintense in relation to liver on T2-weighted image	Markedly hyperintense in relation to liver on T2-weighted image	Hyperintense in relation to liver on T2-weighted image
Necrosis, hemorrhage, or calcifications	Rare	Common	Hemorrhage and cystic areas common	Occasional hemorrhage and cystic areas
Growth rate	Usually stable over time or very slow (<1 cm per year)	Usually rapid (>2 cm per year)	Usually slow (0.5 cm to 1.0 cm per year)	Variable, slow to rapid

Adapted from: Young WF. The incidentally discovered adrenal mass. NEJM. 2007;365:601-10

will not. If unenhanced CT or CSI is indeterminate, contrast enhanced CT with washouts at 10 to 15 minutes has been shown to have excellent sensitivity and specificity, approaching 100%, in differentiating between adenomas and nonadenomatous incidentalomas.

- Characteristics of pheochromocytoma and malignant processes include size (>3 cm), attenuation of >10 HU on unenhanced CT, heterogeneous texture and increased vascularity with decreased contrast washout at 10–15 minutes.

Q. 4 What is the role of functional studies in the evaluation of adrenal incidentaloma?

Ans. Functional imaging studies are mainly performed in patients with biochemical evidence of adrenal, cortical, and medullary hyper secretion to assist surgical planning. Chemical shift imaging on MRI also reflects the lipid content of tissues, with lipid-rich adenomas losing signal intensity on out-of-phase images. In patients with suspected metastasis, 18-fluoro-2-deoxy-d-glucose positron emission tomography has high sensitivity for malignancy but is not specific. A more recently developed ligand, 11C-metomidate, detects non-necrotic adrenocortical tumors (benign and malignant) and is negative in other masses.

CASE 2

A 40-year-old male is subjected to ultrasound examination of the abdomen as he sustained blunt trauma to the abdomen after a road traffic accident. He was healthy till date with no history of hypertension or diabetes. The imaging shows a 6 cm × 5 cm × 4 cm mass in the right adrenal region. A CT abdomen is obtained to further evaluate the mass which shows a well capsulated lesion of the same size mentioned, with areas of low attenuation (–20 to –30, close to that of fat) interspersed with areas of higher attenuation value, uniformly enhancing on contrast administration. The radiologist makes a diagnosis of probable adrenomyelolipoma. The patient is told about the detection of a benign lesion in his adrenal gland. When told that he will need serial imaging to monitor the growth rate of the lesion, the patient chooses resection. Histopathology confirms adrenomyelolipoma.

PS – while adrenomyelolipoma is a benign condition, lipid rich adrenocortical carcinoma with imaging characteristics of adrenomyelolipoma have been reported.

Q. 1 What are the symptoms and signs suggestive of adrenal hyperfunction or malignant disease?

Ans. The groups of hyperfunction that can occur in a patient with adrenal incidentaloma include Cushing's syndrome (including subclinical), pheochromocytoma, primary hyperaldosteronism and lastly adrenocortical carcinoma. Most of these conditions, have subtle, vague features that can be easily missed with a cursory examination. Every attempt must be made to elicit history and signs suggestive of these in all patients with adrenal incidentaloma.

Cushing's syndrome

Symptoms

- Weight gain with central obesity facial rounding and plethora,
- Easy bruising, thin skin, poor wound healing, purple striae, proximal muscle weakness
- Emotional and cognitive changes (e.g. irritability, spontaneous tearfulness, depression)

- Opportunistic and fungal infections, altered reproductive function, acne, and hirsutism.

Signs
- Hypertension, osteopenia, osteoporosis
- Fasting hyperglycemia, diabetes mellitus
- Hypokalemia, hyperlipidemia, and leukocytosis.

Subclinical Cushing's syndrome
The obvious stigmata of Cushing's syndrome may be absent, but, these patients may have the adverse effects of continuous, endogenous cortisol secretion, including hypertension, obesity, diabetes mellitus, and osteoporosis.

Pheochromocytoma: Patient may be asymptomatic; episodic symptoms may occur in spells (paroxysms).

Symptoms
- Forceful heartbeat, pallor, tremor, headache
- Diaphoresis; spells may be either spontaneous or precipitated by postural change, anxiety, medications, maneuvers that increase intra-abdominal pressure (e.g. change in position, lifting, defecation, exercise).

Signs
- Hypertension (paroxysmal or sustained)
- Orthostatic hypotension, pallor, hypertensive retinopathy grades 1–4, tremor, and fever.

Primary aldosteronism

Symptoms
Nocturia, polyuria, muscle cramps, and palpitations

Signs
- Hypertension, mild or severe
- Hypokalemia and mild hypernatremia.

Adrenocortical carcinoma

Symptoms
- Mass effect (e.g. abdominal pain) and symptoms
- Related to adrenal hypersecretion of cortisol (Cushing's syndrome)
  - Androgens (hirsutism, acne, amenorrhea or oligoamenorrhea, oily skin, and increased libido)
  - Estrogens (gynecomastia)
  - Aldosterone (hypokalemia-related symptoms).

Signs
- Hypertension, osteopenia, osteoporosis, diabetes mellitus
- Hypokalemia, hyperlipidemia, fasting hyperglycemia
- Leukocytosis with relative lymphopenia.

Q. 2 Describe the laboratory evaluation in a patient with adrenal incidentaloma?

Ans. All subjects with an incidentally discovered adrenal mass should be screened for both catecholamine overproduction and hypercortisolism, with the exception of patients with adrenal masses whose imaging characteristics are typical for myelolipomas or adrenal cyst. Adrenomyelolipoma is a rare, benign tumor consisting of mature adipose tissue with variable amounts of hematopoietic elements (Table 13.2).

All patients undergo the following work-up.

- *Electrolytes:* Hypokalemia may suggest hyperaldosteronism; hypokalemia may be present in Cushing's syndrome.
- *Fasting lipid profile:* Hyperlipidemia may be present in Cushing's syndrome.
- *Fasting blood glucose:* Hyperglycemia may be present in Cushing's syndrome or pheochromocytomas

TABLE 13.2 Laboratory evaluation of the patient with adrenal incidentaloma

Possible diagnosis	*Screening test*	*Causes of false positive results*	*Confirmatory tests*
Subclinical Cushing's syndrome	Overnight dexamethasone (1 mg) suppression test; abnormal result: serum cortisol, >1.8 µg per deciliter	Medications that accelerate hepatic metabolism of dexamethasone	Serum corticotropin, cortisol in a blood specimen—2-day low-dose dexamethasone suppression test
Pheochromocytoma	Measurement of fractionated metanephrines and catecholamines in a 24-hr urinary specimen	Any situation (e.g. illness requiring hospitalization) or medication (e.g. tricyclic antidepressant) that increases endogenous production of catecholamines	Iodine-123 metaiodobenzylguanidine scintigraphy, MRI
Primary aldosteronism (In patients with hypertension)	The plasma aldosterone concentration and plasma renin activity ratio of ≥20 and a plasma aldosterone concentration of ≥15 ng per deciliter are positive results	Assay and biologic variability	To confirm the diagnosis of primary aldosteronism: aldosterone suppression testing with either a saline infusion test or 24-hour urinary aldosterone excretion test while the patient maintains a high-sodium diet-adrenal venous sampling should be considered

- Screening test for Cushing's syndrome with late night salivary cortisol or overnight (1 mg) dexamethasone suppression test (OST).
- Screening for pheochromocytoma with fractionated plasma metanephrines.

Patients with HTN should also have plasma renin/aldosterone ratio measured to assess for hyperaldosteronism. If screening for hormonal activity is positive, further testing is indicated to confirm hormonal autonomy.

Subclinical Cushing's syndrome: Best strategy for measurement of autonomous adrenocortical secretion is by an overnight dexamethasone (1 mg) suppression test. The use of a cortisol level greater than 1.8 µg/dL with sensitivity of >95% is standard to define abnormal values according to this test. A cut-off point of 5 µg/dL was associated with a specificity of 100% and a sensitivity of 58% in 1 study, whereas a lower cut-off point of about 1.8 µg/dL had a 75% to 100% sensitivity and a 72% to 82% specificity. Hence, we recommend use of the higher cut-off point (5 µg/dL),which has a higher specificity.

The specificity of the 1 mg overnight dexamethasone suppression test is 91%; if the result is abnormal-confirmatory testing should be performed to rule out a false positive result. Serum cortisol ≥5 µg/dL at 21–23 hours are appropriate diagnostic criteria for SCS.

- *Clinically silent pheochromocytoma:* Measurement of fractionated metanephrines and catecholamines in a 24-hour urine specimen is recommended for all patients with adrenal incidentalomas. Elevated levels of fractionated metanephrines, catecholamines, or both has high sensitivity and specificity for pheochromocytoma.
- *Primary aldosteronism:* Reasonable screening test is the ratio of the ambulatory morning plasma aldosterone concentration to plasma renin activity, If this ratio is high, the diagnosis of primary aldosteronism should be confirmed by an additional measurement of mineralocorticoid secretory autonomy.
- Blood levels of androgens (testosterone and dehydroepiandrosterone sulphate) or estrogens (estradiol) are not routine, but measured when there are signs or symptoms of virilization in women or feminization in men.

CASE 3

A 35-year-old farmer sustains chest injuries following an accident at the farm for which he is subjected to CT imaging of thorax and abdomen which reveals bilateral adrenal mass, measuring 4 cm × 3 cm × 4 cm, homogeneous, smooth walled, isodense with liver and well enhancing on contrast administration. He is asymptomatic prior to the accident. Examination reveals a normally built male, normal vitals, no postural drop in blood pressure. No obvious hyperpigmentation. Biochemical evaluation are all normal except a serum sodium levels of 129 mEq/L. TSH, total T4 levels are normal. At 8 am cortisol is 5 µg/dL with a corresponding ACTH of 100 pg/mL. A synacthen stimulation test with 250 µg given IV is done and 60 min cortisol of 13 µg/dL is obtained. A diagnosis of Addison's disease is made. Chest X-ray and Mantoux test are normal. 24-hour urine collection for metanephrines is normal. A CT-guided FNAC is performed which reveals 2–4 μm oval, budding yeast forms with a probable diagnosis of histoplasmosis. ELISA for human immunodeficiency virus is negative. Patient is started on hydrocortisone 15 mg/day in two split doses. Patient is given intravenous amphotericin B for two weeks followed by oral itraconazole for one year.

Q. 1 What is the role of fine needle biopsy ?

Ans. Fine-needle biopsy (FNB) is currently not recommended for the routine work-up of AI. Often, clinical, hormonal and radiologic findings can effectively direct treatment. Infectious diseases form an important reason for FNA, especially in our country as illustrated in case 2. It is also associated with relatively rare, but significant complications; pheochromocytoma must always be ruled out before biopsy is undertaken to avoid potentially life-threatening hemorrhage and hypertensive crisis.

Q. 2 What is the risk of malignant transformation of an adrenal incidentaloma?

Ans. Risk of malignant transformation of an untreated adrenal incidentaloma, qualified as a benign lesion, subsequently developing malignancy appears to be very low. In patients with adrenal incidentalomas, followed up for an average of 4 years, 5–20% showed mass enlargement >1 cm and/or appearance of another mass in the contralateral gland.

Q. 3 What is the risk of evolution toward overt hypersecretion?

Ans. Development of overt Cushing's syndrome during the follow-up was observed in <1% of cases, whereas appearance of silent biochemical alterations was reported in a 0–11% cases across different studies. Masses of 3 cm or greater are more likely to develop silent hyperfunction than smaller tumors, and the risk seems to plateau after 3–4 years.

The onset of catecholamine overproduction or hyperaldosteronism during long-term follow-up is very rare.

Q. 4 What is the morbidity and mortality of subclinical Cushing syndrome ?

Ans. An increased frequency of hypertension, central obesity, impaired glucose tolerance or diabetes, hyperlipidemia and osteoporosis has been described in patients with subclinical Cushing syndrome in a number of retrospective or cross-sectional studies.

Despite the reported association between SCS and the metabolic syndrome, evidence of increased mortality in patients who have clinically inapparent adrenal adenomas and subclinical Cushing syndrome is lacking. The (scarce) available data suggest that most patients with adrenal incidentalomas remain asymptomatic throughout life. Also, long-term follow-up data in unavailable to choose surgery over medical management. The AACE/AAES Medical Guidelines for the management of adrenal incidentalomas suggest that until further evidence is available regarding the long-term benefits of adrenalectomy,surgical resection should be reserved for those with worsening of hypertension, abnormal glucose tolerance, dyslipidemia, or osteoporosis especially younger patients.

CASE 4

A 42-year-old woman is subjected to computed tomography (CT) scan of the abdomen for recurrent complaints of epigastric discomfort which revealed a 2.6 cm × 2 cm × 3 cm well rounded mass in her left adrenal gland, with a attenuation value of 5 HU, well enhancing on contrast administration. Washout study is not done. She was diagnosed with hypertension and diabetes since 2 years for which she is on amlodipine 5 mg/day and metformin 2 g/day. She has progressively gained weight since the birth of her last child birth ten years ago and currently is obese with a BMI 28 kg/m^2. Her menstrual cycles are irregular since 5 years and bleeds every 2 months only after ingestion of a pill taken twice daily for a week. On examination, central obesity is present, supraclavicular areas are full. Skin appears normal with no thinning, bruising or striae. No proximal myopathy or hirsutism is noted.

Management: The imaging characteristics indicate a benign lesion. Her clinical profile validates screening for pheochromocytoma, Cushing's syndrome and primary hyperaldosteronism. All her tests are negative. She is advised to follow-up every 6 months with repeat imaging and biochemical testing.

Q. 1 What is the management of adrenal incidentaloma?

Ans.

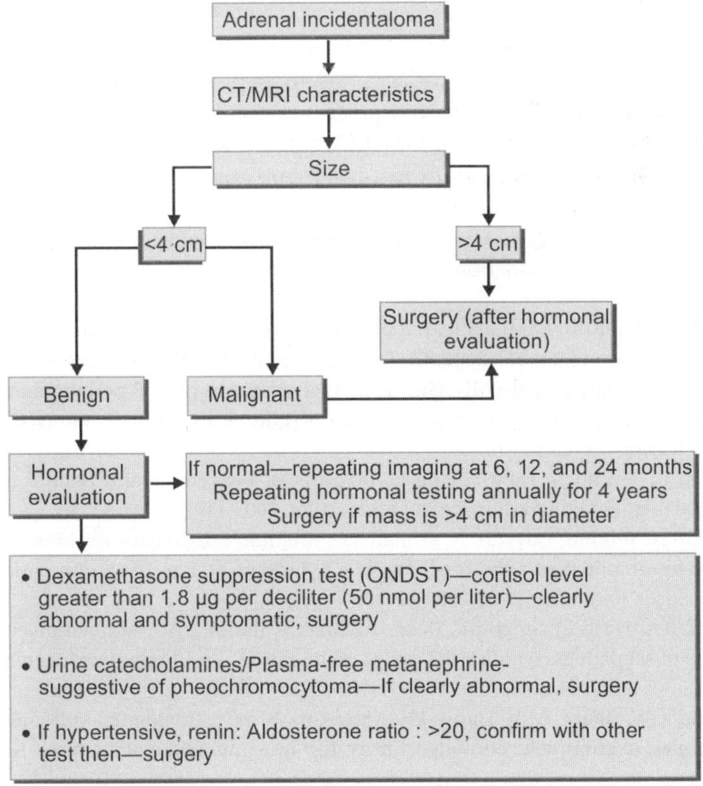

Q. 2 How to perform follow-up in adrenal incidentalomas?

Ans.

- There is no consensus on appropriate follow-up evaluation for those who do not have surgery, and one must be guided by clinical evaluation and radiological diagnosis of the mass. After initial diagnostic evaluation, follow-up of adrenal incidentalomas includes imaging evaluation at 6–12 months to assess for mass enlargement.
- For lesions that do not increase in size, further radiological follow-up is not required. Biochemical testing annually (overnight 1 mg dexamethasone suppression test and fractionated plasma metanephrines) are done yearly for 4 years to exclude emergence of subclinical hormonal hypersecretion.
- Patients with an adrenal incidentaloma are at risk for tumor growth and development of hormonal alterations. A long-term follow-up study (12–120 months, median 25.5 months) of 64 patients with incidental adrenal masses revealed that cumulative risk of developing endocrine abnormalities was 17% at 1 year, 29% at 2 years, and 47% at 5 years; cumulative risk of mass enlargement was 6% at 1 year, 14% at 2 years, and 29% at 5 years.
- Patients with laboratory features of cortisol excess should be screened at annual intervals and recommended annual biochemical screening for catecholamine and cortisol excess for 4 years.

SUGGESTED READING

1. Alexander CM, Landsman PB, Teutsch SM, Haffner SM. NCEP defined metabolic syndrome, diabetes, and prevalence of coronary heart disease among NHANES III participants age 50 years and older, Third National Health and Nutrition Examination Survey (NHANES III); National Cholesterol Education Program (NCEP). Diabetes. 2003;52:1210-4. (doi:10.2337/diabetes.52.5.1210)
2. Angeli A, Osella G, Ali A, Terzolo M. Adrenal incidentaloma: an overview of clinical and epidemiological data from the National Italian Study Group. Horm Res. 1997;47: 279-83.
3. Angeli A, Terzolo M. Adrenal incidentaloma - a modern disease with old complications. J Clin Endocrinol Metabol. 2002;87:4869-71. (doi:10.1210/jc.2002- 021436).
4. Arellano RS, Harisinghani MG, Gervais DA, et al. Image-guided percutaneous biopsy of the adrenal gland: review of indications, technique, and complications. Curr Probl Diagn Radiol. 2003;32:3-10.
5. Barzon L, Sonino N, Fallo F, Palù G, Boscaro M. Prevalence and natural history of adrenal incidentalomas. European J Endocrinol. 2003;149:273-85.
6. Benitah N, Yeh BM, Qayyum A, Williams G, Breiman RS, Coakley FV. Minor morphologic abnormalities of adrenal glands at CT: prognostic importance in patients with lung cancer. Radiology. 2005;235:517-22.
7. Bhansali A, Dash RJ, Singh SK, Behra A, Singh P, Radotra BD. Adrenal myelolipoma: profile of six patients with a brief review of literature. Int J Endocrinol Metab. 2003;1: 33-40.
8. Boland GW, Blake MA, Hahn PF, Mayo-Smith WW. Incidental adrenal lesions: principles, techniques, and algorithms for imaging characterization. Radiology. 2008;249:756-75.

9. Caoili EM, Korobkin M, Francis IR, et al. Adrenal masses: characterization with combined unenhanced and delayed enhanced CT. Radiology. 2002;222:629-33.
10. Emral R, Uysal AR, Asik M, et al. Prevalence of subclinical Cushing's syndrome in 70 patients with adrenal incidentaloma: clinical, biochemical and surgical outcomes. Endocr J. 2003;50:399-408.
11. Grossrubatscher E, Vignati F, Possa M, Loli P. The natural history of incidentally discovered adrenocortical adenomas: a retrospective evaluation. J Endocrinol Invest. 2001;24:846-55.
12. Herra MF, Pantoja JP, Espagna N. Adrenal incidentalomas. In: Linos D, van Heerden JA (Eds). Adrenal Glands: Diagnostic Aspects and Surgical Therapy. Berlin: Springer-Verlag; 2005. pp.231-44.
13. Kawaguchi K, Kuwa K, Takatsu A, Tani W, Kobayashi T. Standarization of cortisol measurement and results of technical examination of low range of cortisol measurement. ACTH Related Peptides. 2012;22:2-8 (In Japanese).
14. Lal G, Duh QY. Laparoscopic adrenalectomy—indications and technique. Surgical Oncology. 2003;12:105-23. (doi:10.1016/ S0960-7404(03)00036-7).
15. Libè R, Dall'Asta C, Barbetta L, Baccarelli A, Beck-Peccoz P, Ambrosi B. Long-term follow-up study of patients with adrenal incidentalomas. European J Endocrinol. 2002;147:489-94.
16. Lynette K, Nieman. Approach to patient with an Adrenal Incidentaloma. J Clin Endocrinol Metab. 2010;95(9):4106-13.
17. Mansmann G, Lau J, Balk E, Rothberg M, Miyachi Y, Bornstein SR. The clinically inapparent adrenal mass: update in diagnosis and management. Endocrine Reviews. 2004;25:309-40. (doi:10.1210/er.2002-0031).
18. Mulatero P, Stowasser M, Loh KC, et al. Increased diagnosis of primary aldosteronism, including surgically correctable forms, in centers from five continents. J Clin Endocrinol Metab. 2004;89:1045-50.
19. Nieman LK, Biller BM, Findling JW, Newell-Price J, Savage MO, et al. The diagnosis of Cushing's syndrome: An Endocrine Society Clinical Practice Guideline. J Clin Endocrinol Metab. 2008;93:1526-40.
20. Rossi R, Tauchmanova L, Luciano A, et al. Subclinical Cushing's syndrome in patients with adrenal incidentaloma: clinical and biochemical features. J Clin Endocrinol Metab. 2000;85:1440-8.
21. Sawka AM, Jaeschke R, Singh RJ, Young WF Jr. A comparison of biochemical tests for pheochromocytoma: measurement of fractionated plasma metanephrines compared with the combination of 24-hour urinary metanephrines and catecholamines. J Clin Endocrinol Metab. 2003;88:553-8.
22. Tauchmanova L, Rossi R, Biondi B, et al. Patients with subclinical Cushing's syndrome due to adrenal adenoma have increased cardiovascular risk. J Clin Endocrinol Metab. 2002;87:4872-8.
23. Terzolo M, Bovio S, Reimondo G, Pia A, Osella G, Borretta G, et al. Subclinical Cushing's syndrome in adrenal incidentalomas. Endocrinology and Metabolism Clinics of North America. 2005;34:423-39.
24. Young WF. Management approaches to adrenal incidentalomas. Aview from Rochester, Minnesota. Endocrinology and Metabolism Clinics of North America. 2000;29:159-85. (doi:10.1016/ S0889-8529(05)70122-5).
25. Zeiger MA, Thompson GB, Duh QY, Hamrahian AH, Angelos P, Elaraj D, Fishman E, Kharlip J. The American Association of Clinical Endocrinologists and American Association of Endocrine Surgeons medical guidelines for the management of adrenal incidentalomas. Endocrine Practice. 2009;15:1-20.

CHAPTER

14

Approach to Amenorrhea

Pramila Kalra

CASE 1

A 25-year-old unmarried girl comes to the endocrinology OPD with history of amenorrhea for past 7 months. Her menarche happened at the age of 13 years. She has no other complaints except for mild lethargy or fatigue. She has no known endocrinological problem. She complains of some occasional episodes of sweating and palpitations. She has no complaints of headache or any visual disturbances. She has no complaints of vomiting or any change in weight. She does not give any history of any drug intake. She has not taken any treatment for amenorrhea till now. She has not undergone any gynecological procedures till now. Prior to seven months, her menses were regular. Her mother is concerned about her amenorrhea as she is getting married next month and her future conception prospects.

Her height is 160 cm and her predicted height is 158 cm. Her weight is 60 kg. She has normal secondary sexual characters development.

She has no features of virilization. She has no similar history in the family and she has no hirsutism or acne. She has no galactorrhea.

Q. 1 What is secondary amenorrhea?

Ans. Secondary amenorrhea is defined as the cessation of previously regular menses for three months or the cessation of previously irregular menses for six months.

Q. 2 What are the causes of secondary amenorrhea?

Ans. The most common cause is pregnancy followed by polycystic ovarian syndrome.

Acquired causes like Asherman's syndrome (intrauterine synechiae),cervical stenosis, primary ovarian insufficiency, gonadal dysgenesis other than Turner's syndrome or Turner syndrome variant, autoimmune destruction, chemotherapy or radiation, disease of the pituitary ranging from autoimmune hypophysitis to non-functioning and functioning pituitary adenomas., empty sella syndrome, hyperprolactinemia, use of drugs like cocaine to pituitary infiltrative disorders, medications like antidepressants, antihistaminics, antipsychotics and opiates. Hypothalamic causes like eating disorders stress, traumatic brain injury, androgen excess causes including androgen secreting tumors.

Most cases of secondary amenorrhea can be attributed to polycystic ovary syndrome, hypothalamic amenorrhea, hyperprolactinemia, or primary ovarian insufficiency.

Q. 3 What is the first step in the evaluation of this patient?

Ans. Any woman who comes with secondary amenorrhea a pregnancy test is mandatory and has to be done as the first diagnostic test.

Measurement of serum beta subunit of human chorionic gonadotropin (hCG) is the most sensitive test. Even if the home pregnancy test is negative and pregnancy is suspected a serum testing for beta subunit of hCG should be done.

The pregnancy test is negative in this patient.

Q. 4 What is the next step in making the diagnosis?

Ans. Before proceeding on to the full battery of tests any precipitating factor for hypothalamic amenorrhea or any other cause of amenorrhea has to be elicited in the history.

To elicit the history if lately there has been any stress, change in weight, diet or exercise habits, or illness that might result in hypothalamic amenorrhea (HA).

Is the woman taking any drugs that might cause or be associated with amenorrhea? The drug might have been taken for a systemic illness that can itself cause hypothalamic amenorrhea. If the patient is on any contraceptives or has recently discontinued them which can be associated with several months of amenorrhea.

Ingestion of androgenic drugs or high-dose progestin can cause amenorrhea. Intake of drugs which increase serum prolactin concentrations should also be carefully looked for in the records.

If the women complain of acne, hirsutism, or deepening of the voice it can be a pointer towards testosterone excess state ranging from polycystic ovary syndrome to increased androgen production because of the tumor.

If the patient has symptoms suggestive of hypothalamic—or pituitary disease, including headaches, visual field defects, fatigue, or polyuria and polydipsia.

If the patient has symptoms of estrogen deficiency, including hot flashes, vaginal dryness, poor sleep, or decreased libido and may point towards ovarian insufficiency.

An exception is women with hypothalamic amenorrhea who do not usually have these symptoms despite the presence of similarly low serum estrogen concentrations.

Any history of postpartum hemorrhage and failure of lactation may point towards a possibility of Sheehan's syndrome.

History and examination of a patient with secondary amenorrhea (important points)

- Exercise, weight loss, chronic illness—pointers towards hypothalamic amenorrhea
- History of any drug use like oral contraceptive pills or injectable hormonal therapy
- History of any previous chemotherapy or radiation exposure
- Previous pelvic radiation
- Vasomotor symptoms-premature ovarian failure
- BMI—can help in diagnosing PCOS (though they can be lean also)
- Acne, hirsutism-suggest hyperandrogenemia and all relevant causes to be ruled out
- Virilization—can point towards androgen or ovarian tumors or congenital adrenal hyperplasia or ovarian hyperthecosis
- If BMI very low <18 kg/m^2—can point towards eating disorders like anorexia nervosa
- Acanthosis nigricans, skin tags—markers of insulin resistance
- Breast examination for galactorrhea
- Vulvovaginal examination—to look for signs of estrogen deficiency
- Parotid gland swelling or dental enamel erosion—bulimia
- Primary hypothyroidism or hyperthyroidism—signs and symptoms
- Any markers of Cushing's syndrome
- Symptoms suggestive of any pituitary tumor or pathology.

Q. 5 What battery of tests is required?

Ans. A complete blood cell count, urinalysis, and serum chemistries should be evaluated to help rule out systemic disease. Serum prolactin, FSH, estradiol, and thyrotropin levels and prolactin should also be measured routinely in the initial evaluation of amenorrhea once pregnancy has been excluded. The levels of androgens also need to be checked which includes serum testosterone, DHEAS and also 17 hydroxy progesterone.

Q. 6 What do these tests tell us?

Ans. If the prolactin level is high it may point towards a pituitary tumor secreting prolactin only if the levels are beyond 200 ng/mL. A level between 10 and 200 ng/mL is a borderline range. In all cases drug history should be elicited to rule out any drug induced hyperprolactinemia. Psychotropic drugs, hypothyroidism, stress, and meals can also raise prolactin levels.

An FSH level of more than 40 mIU/mL shows premature ovarian failure and has to be confirmed after one month with a repeat testing.

LH levels can be elevated in cases of 17,20 lyase deficiency, 17-hydroxylase deficiency, and premature ovarian failure.

LH levels can vary from 50 to 400 pg/mL depending on the early follicular to preovulatory estradiol surge.

In menopausal women the levels are typically less than 20 pg/mL.

Amenorrhea is an uncommon presentation of thyroid disorders but TSH and T4 levels are to be done to rule out hyperthyroidism or hypothyroidism.

The levels of androgens like testosterone and DHEAS point towards any cause of hyperandrogenemia leading to amenorrhea.

Her hormonal evaluation shows FSH level of 60 IU/L.

Her serum E2 level is 20 pg/mL.

Her TSH, T4 is in normal range.

Her prolactin level is 20 ng/mL.

Her serum testosterone is 30 ng/mL.

A diagnosis of premature ovarian failure is made and she is counselled about need of hormonal therapy.

Q. 7 What is premature ovarian failure?

Ans. Premature ovarian failure (POF) is an early ovarian malfunction different from menopause, which disturbs production of follicles resulting in amenorrhea under the age of 40 in 1–3% of reproductive age women. About 10–28% of the patients experience primary amenorrhea and about 4–18% show secondary amenorrhea. Affected women show menstrual problems followed by an elevated level of gonadotropins [follicle stimulating hormone (FSH) ≥40 IU/L] and hypoestrogenism for an average four months.

Q. 8 Are all patients with premature ovarian failure infertile?

Ans. All patients may not be infertile as they may have unpredictable ovarian function. About 75% of women with 46,XX spontaneous primary ovarian insufficiency have potentially functional graafian follicles remaining in the ovary. Inappropriate follicle luteinization is the most common pathophysiologic mechanism that prevents ovulation and pregnancy in these women.

Q. 9 What is the likely etiology of premature ovarian failure?

Ans. The likely etiologies include infection, autoimmune disorders and metabolic factors are likely responsible for the disorder development. In 90% of observed cases, the etiology is unknown and the disease is defined as idiopathic POF.

Q. 10 What are the genetic associations of the disease?

Ans. Most POF cases are sporadic and it is suggested that between 4% and 31% of them are familial and abnormalities of the X chromosome are presented as the most important causes of the disease followed by the fragile X mental retardation (FMR1) premutation which is present in POF patients with frequencies of 13 and 6%, respectively. Loss of one X chromosome as X monosomy [Turner syndrome (TS)], the related gene deletions and X/autosome translocations, trisomy X, X linked gene mutations and premutations and anomalies of autosomal linked genes have been widely studied in correlation with POF disease.

The lady in the case is put on estrogen and progesterone combination and is told to follow-up after 3 months.

Q. 11 Do we need to screen her for any other endocrine organs?

Ans. Yes because she has premature ovarian failure so she may be having other endocrine involvement so anti-TPO titer and a 8 am serum cortisol level need to be tested and we have to watch for development of any other endocrine organ involvement in future.

Q. 12 What is Perrault syndrome?

Ans. Perrault syndrome is characterized by sensorineural hearing loss (SNHL) in males and females, and ovarian dysfunction in females. The SNHL is bilateral and ranges in severity from moderate with early-childhood onset to profound with prelingual (congenital) onset to moderate with early-childhood onset. When onset is in early childhood, hearing loss can be progressive. Ovarian dysfunction ranges from gonadal dysgenesis (absent or streak gonads) manifesting as primary amenorrhea to primary ovarian insufficiency (POI) defined as cessation of menses before age 40 years. Fertility in affected males is reported as normal (although the number of reported males is limited). Neurologic features described in some affected women include developmental delay or intellectual disability, cerebellar ataxia, and motor and sensory peripheral neuropathy.

Q. 13 What are the recommendations for treatment of patient with premature ovarian failure?

Ans. Estrogen-progestin replacement therapy is recommended for prevention of osteoporosis in women with primary ovarian insufficiency. An additional benefit of symptomatic control of vasomotor symptoms and vaginal dryness is provided and possibly there is an additional benefit on the prevention of heart disease.

Q. 14 Up to what age hormone therapy is recommended for women with premature ovarian failure?

Ans. The premenopausal hormone therapy can be continued in the absence of any other contraindications until approximately age 52 years, the average age of natural menopause.

Q. 15 Is there any benefit of androgen therapy in these women?

Ans. No there is no proven benefit in women with normal adrenal function.

Q. 16 What are the options of hormone therapy?

Ans. Cyclic treatment with both estrogen and progesterone (in view of intact uterus in many POF patients and to prevent endometrial hyperplasia and neoplasia that can result with treatment of estrogen alone.

Estrogen (e.g. micronized estradiol 1–2 mg daily or conjugated equine estrogens 0.625–1.25 mg daily) or transdermal treatment regimens (0.1 mg/24 hours). Progestogen (e.g. micronized progesterone 200 mg daily or medroxyprogesterone acetate 10 mg daily for 12–14 days each month).

Q. 17 What is the pathophysiology of amenorrhea in athletes?

Ans. Due to decreased energy availability in athletes there is decrease in fat mass, and alterations in adipokines (such as leptin and adiponectin) and fat-regulated hormones (such as ghrelin and peptide YY). These hormones impact the HPG axis in animal models, and it is possible that in athletes alterations in fat-related hormones signal the state of energy availability to the hypothalamus and contribute to suppression of gonadotropin pulsatility, hypothalamic amenorrhea and consequent decreased BMD.

CASE 2

A girl is brought at the age of 17 years with complaints of primary amenorrhea. She is born at full term with no perinatal complications and her motor and sensory milestones are normal. She is 165 cm in height and her predicted height is 155 cm. On examination she has B3 staging of breast with absence of axillary and pubic hairs. Her serum E2 level is low and her FSH and LH are high. Her serum testosterone is 1000 ng/mL and her USG pelvis does not show any uterus or ovaries. She has a blind vaginal pouch on vaginal examination by the gynecologist.

Q. 1 What is primary amenorrhea?

Ans Primary amenorrhea is defined as the absence of menses at age 15 years in the presence of normal growth and secondary sexual characteristics. Some authorities recommend evaluating a girl for primary amenorrhea if her menses have not occurred by age 15 years. If no menses have occurred and there is an absence of secondary sexual characteristics, such as breast development, evaluation for primary amenorrhea should be done at the age of 13 years (Flowchart 14.1).

Q. 2 What is the probable diagnosis in her case?

Ans. In view of the high serum testosterone with a female phenotype with poorly developed secondary sexual characteristics a diagnosis of complete androgen sensitivity syndrome is made and a karyotyping is done.

The karyotype shows XY and so the diagnosis of complete androgen insensitivity is confirmed

Q. 3 What are the points in favor of the diagnosis?

Ans. Female phenotype with normal breast development

- Primary amenorrhea
- Little or no axillary or pubic hair
- Absent uterus, but testes present

FLOWCHART 14.1 Approach to a case of amenorrhea

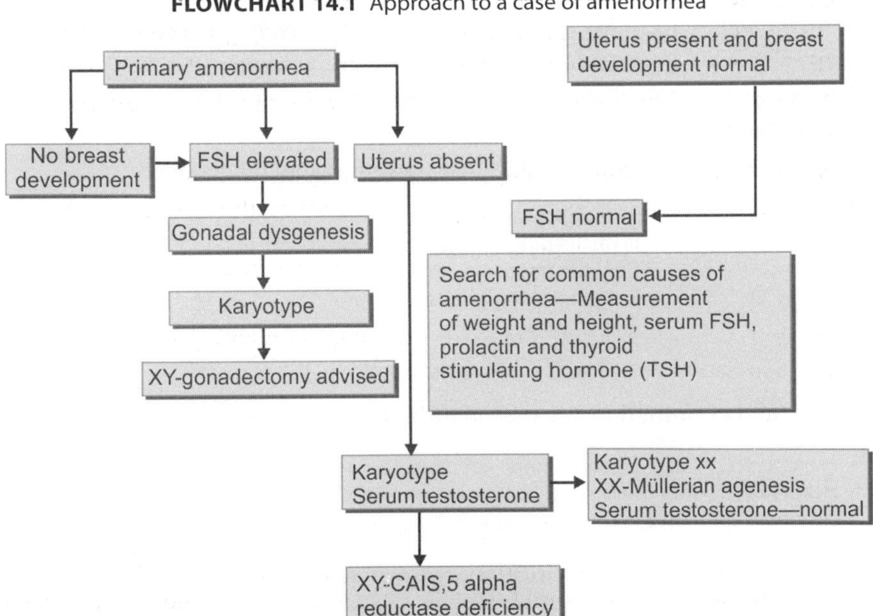

- 46,XY karyotype
- Blind vaginal pouch on exam
- Serum testosterone concentrations in the normal adult male range.

Q. 4 What is the next step in this patient?

Ans. The next step in the evaluation is to search for testis intra-abdominally. A MRI is done which shows intra-abdominal testis in the iliac fossa and a gonadectomy is planned.

Q. 5 When should gonadectomy be done in CAIS?

Ans. Girls with CAIS have a normal pubertal growth spurt and feminize at the time of expected puberty (secondary to aromatization of androgen to estrogen), and testicular tumors do not usually develop until after this time. Therefore, gonadectomy in women with CAIS is typically delayed until sexual maturation is complete. This approach also respects patient autonomy. However, in some situations, the convenience of combining gonadectomy with hernia repair or the need to relieve symptoms of discomfort from labial or inguinal testes justifies removal of the testes before puberty.

Q. 6 What hormone therapy should be offered to this patient?

Ans. The patient first needs to be counseled and after patient's consent first gonadectomy has to be done and the patient has to be continued on adult dose of estrogens.

If the gonadectomy is performed before puberty for some reason the puberty induction protocol for estrogen therapy has to be followed.

Q. 7 What other treatment should be done for her?

Ans. In patients with subnormal vaginal depth a dilator therapy may be done prior to the time when an active sex life is contemplated, and vaginoplasty should be undertaken only in those women who do not have an adequate response to dilator therapy.

Q. 8 What should be the sex of rearing in this patient as she is a genetic male but a phenotypic female?

Ans. The sex of rearing would be female but she would be infertile.

Physiological amenorrhea
- Breastfeeding
- Contraception
- Exogenous androgens
- Menopause
- Pregnancy

History and examination in a case of primary amenorrhea (important points)

- Exercise, weight loss, chronic illness—pointers towards hypothalamic amenorrhea
- History of any drug use like oral contraceptive pills or injectable hormonal therapy
- History of any previous chemotherapy or radiation exposure
- Previous pelvic radiation
- History of menarche and menstrual history in mother and sisters

- Evaluation of pubertal development
- Height
- Weight
- Arm span (normal arm span for adults is within 5 cm of height)
- Cyclic abdominal pain—outflow tract obstruction
- Examination—hirsutism, acne, striae, increased pigmentation over the skin—could point towards causes of hyperandrogenemia like PCOS, Cushing's syndrome, hyperprolactenemia
- Evaluation for the classic physical features of Turner syndrome such as low hair line, web neck, shield chest, and widely spaced nipples should be noted. These patients mostly have short stature
- Anosmia-can be a pointer towards Kallman's syndrome
- Symptoms and signs suggestive of hypothyroidism or hyperthyroidism
- An assessment of breast development (e.g. by Tanner staging) and also for galactorrhea
- Gonads presenting as inguinal hernia-androgen insensitivity syndrome
- Genital examination—clitoral size to see for any evidence of clitoromegaly, pubertal hair development, intactness of the hymen, depth of the vagina, and presence of a cervix, uterus, and ovaries
- If the vagina cannot be penetrated with a finger, rectal examination may allow evaluation of the internal organs
- Pelvic ultrasound is also useful to determine the presence or absence of Müllerian structures
- Symptoms and signs—suggestive of Cushing's syndrome
- Features of anorexia nervosa or bulimia-hypothalamic amenorrhea
- Symptoms suggestive of any pituitary tumor or pathology
- To see for any gonads presenting as inguinal hernias

A Detailed History Including

1. Patient's height relative to other family members—Short stature may indicate Turner syndrome or hypothalamic-pituitary disease.
2. History of whether patient has passed through all stages of puberty—Lack of pubertal development suggests ovarian or pituitary failure or a chromosomal abnormality.
3. Is there a family history of delayed or absent puberty—Suggesting a possible familial disorder, CDGP.
4. Neonatal crisis of diarrhea, shock, electrolyte imbalance—Suggests congenital adrenal hyperplasia.
5. History suggestive of any chronic disease.
6. History suggestive of PCOS which can present as primary amenorrhea with hirsutism
7. The presence of virilization—Point towards an androgen-secreting ovarian or adrenal tumor, or the presence of Y chromosome material.
8. History of stress, change in weight, diet, or exercise habits, or illness that might result in hypothalamic amenorrhea. Any drugs that might cause or be associated with amenorrhea—the medication may be taken for a systemic illness that itself can cause hypothalamic amenorrhea (e.g. sarcoidosis). Alternatively, drugs such as heroin and methadone can alter hypothalamic gonadotropin secretion.
9. History of galactorrhea (suggestive of excess prolactin).

SUGGESTED READING

1. Fourman LT, Fazeli PK. Neuroendocrine causes of amenorrhea—an update. J Clin Endocrinol Metab. 2015;100(3):812-24. doi: 10.1210/jc.2014-3344. Epub 2015 Jan 12. Review.
2. Golden NH, Carlson JL. The pathophysiology of amenorrhea in the adolescent. Ann N Y Acad Sci. 2008;1135:163-78. doi: 10.1196/annals.1429.014. Review.
3. Goswami D, Conway GS. Premature ovarian failure. Horm Res. 2007;68(4):196-202. Epub 2007 May 9. Review.
4. Hall JE. Polycystic ovarian disease as a neuroendocrine disorder of the female reproductive axis. Endocrinol Metab Clin North Am. 1993;22(1):75-92. Review.
5. Helling AN. Premature ovarian failure. Reproduction. 2010;140(5):633-41: 10.1530/REP-09-0567. Epub 2010 Aug 17. Review.
6. Klein DA, Poth MA. Amenorrhea: an approach to diagnosis and management. Am Fam Physician. 2013;87(11):781-8. Review
7. Majumdar A, Mangal NS. Hyperprolactinemia. J Hum Reprod Sci. 2013;6(3):168-75.
8. Misra M, Klibanski A. Endocrine consequences of anorexia nervosa. Lancet Diabetes Endocrinol. 2014;2(7):581-92. doi: 10.1016/S2213-8587(13)70180-3.Epub 2014 Apr 2. Review.
9. Mitan LA. Menstrual dysfunction in anorexia nervosa. J Pediatr Adolesc Gynecol. 2004;17(2):81-5. Review.
10. Newman WG, Friedman TB, Conway GS. Perrault Syndrome. 2014. In: Pagon RA, Adam MP, Ardinger HH, Wallace SE, Amemiya A, Bean LJH, Bird TD, Dolan CR, Fong CT, Smith RJH, Stephens K (Eds). GeneReviews® [Internet]. Seattle (WA):University of Washington, Seattle; 1993-2015.
11. Oupas ND, Georgopoulos NA. Menstrual function in sports. Hormones (Athens). 2011;10(2):104-16. Review.
12. Pouresmaeili F, Fazeli Z. Premature ovarian failure: a critical condition in the reproductive potential with various genetic causes. Int J Fertil Steril. 2014;8(1):1-12. Epub 2014 Mar 9. Review.Int J Fertil Steril. 2014;8(1):1-12.
13. Russell M, Misra M. Influence of ghrelin and adipocytokines on bone mineral density in adolescent female athletes with amenorrhea and eumenorrheic athletes. Med Sport Sci. 2010;55:103-13. doi: 10.1159/000321975. Epub 2010 Oct 14. Review.
14. Shah D, Nagarajan N. Premature menopause —Meeting the needs. Post ReprodHealth. 2014;20(2):62-68. [Epub ahead of print] Review.
15. Silva CA, Yamakami LY, Aikawa NE, Araujo DB, Carvalho JF, Bonfá E. Autoimmune primary ovarian insufficiency. Autoimmun Rev. 2014;13(4-5):427-30. doi:10.1016/j.autrev. 2014.01.003. Epub 2014 Jan 10. Review.
16. Skorupskaite K, George JT, Anderson RA. The kisspeptin-GnRH pathway in human reproductive health and disease. Hum Reprod Update. 2014;20(4):485-500. doi: 10.1093/humupd/dmu009. Epub 2014 Mar 9. Review.

CHAPTER

15

Approach to Hypocalcemia

Pramila Kalra, Neeraj Garg

CASE 1

An 8-year-old girl is brought with complaints of short stature and recurrent seizures. She was started on antiepileptics about 6 months back but 2 days back she developed tetany and her serum calcium was found to be 5 mg/dL and is hence referred to endocrinology. Her calcium levels at the time of seizures were not checked in the past. She is conscious and oriented at the time of examination. Her pulse rate is 110/min and BP is 90/60 mm Hg and respiratory rate is 20/min; she is afebrile. She has moon facies and alopecia. Her BMI is normal, and secondary sexual characteristics are well-developed. There are no bony deformities in the limbs. Signs of latent tetany (Chvostek and Trousseau signs) are positive. There are bilateral cataracts but no evidence of papilledema. Examination of other systems namely cardiovascular, respiratory, and nervous is normal. Emergency investigations show low total serum calcium of 5 mg/dL (8.5–10.5 mg/dL) and her ionized calcium is 2.5 mg/dL (4.60–5.30 mg/dL). Serum magnesium level (1.5 mg/dL) is low normal and her phosphorus is 8 mg/dL (2.5–4.90 mg/dL) and her parathormone is 500 pg/mL (range 11 to 79.5 pg/mL). A noncontrast (NCCT) scan of the brain reveals bilateral basal ganglia and pineal gland calcification. The QTc interval is prolonged to 0.46 seconds.

A provisional diagnosis of hypocalcemic seizures is made.

Q. 1 What is hypocalcemia?

Ans. Hypocalcemia is defined as serum calcium level of less than 8.5 mg/dL. Clinical signs and symptoms are observed when the serum ionized calcium concentration goes below the normal range of ionized calcium.

Hypocalcemia is the hallmark of hypoparathyroidism, which may be inherited either as an isolated endocrinopathy or as part of an autoimmune polyendocrinopathy–candidiasis–ectodermal dystrophy or the DiGeorge syndrome.

Q. 2 What are the causes of hypocalcemia?

Ans. It includes parathyroid related disorders, vitamin D-related disorders and other causes.

Q. 3 What are the parathyroid related disorders causes of hypocalcemia?

Ans. It includes absence of parathyroid gland, congenital cause of absent parathyroid include DiGeorge syndrome, X-linked or autosomally inherited hypoparathyroidism, autoimmune polyglandular syndrome type 1, PTH gene mutations, postsurgical hypoparathyroidism, infiltrative disorders of the parathyroid like hemochromatosis, Wilsons disease, metastasis, hypoparathyroidism following radioactive iodine ablation of the thyroid gland, impaired secretion of the PTH because of hypomagnesemia, respiratory alkalosis and activating mutations of the calcium sensing receptor or target organ resistance because of hypomagnesemia or pseudohypoparathyroidism type 1 or 2.

Q. 4 What are the vitamin D-related disorders?

Ans. They include vitamin D deficiency because of dietary deficiency, inadequate exposure to sunlight or malabsorption. Any accelerated loss of vitamin D due to increased enterohepatic circulation, anticonvulsant medications, impaired hydroxylation of vitamin D due to isoniazid therapy or liver disease, impaired 1 α hydroxylation due to renal disease, vitamin D resistant rickets type 1, oncogenic osteomalacia, target organ resistance, vitamin D resistant rickets type 2 and phenytoin.

Q. 5 What are the other causes?

Ans. The other causes include Hungry bone syndrome, osteoblastic malignancies, babies born to diabetic or hyperparathyroid mother, HIV infection and drug therapy, chelation include foscarnet, phosphate infusion, infusion of citrated blood products, infusion of EDTA containing contrast agents and fluoride, critical illness like pancreatitis and toxic shock syndrome.

Q. 6 What is pseudohypoparathyroidism?

Ans. Pseudohypoparathyroidism is characterized by end-organ resistance to the effects of parathormone. PTH binds to the PTH receptor, which in turn, activates cAMP through guanine nucleotide regulatory proteins (Gs). These proteins consist of alpha, beta, and gamma subunits.

Pseudohypoparathyroidism is classified into types I and II. Type I is further subdivided into 1a, 1b, and 1c.

Q. 7 How to differentiate between the different types of pseudohypoparathyroidism?

Ans. Type 1 a is due to reduction in the Gs-alpha protein. This disorder comprises the biochemical features of hypocalcemia and somatic features of Albright's hereditary osteodystrophy (AHO) which comprises of short stature, obesity, mental retardation, brachymetacarpia and brachymetatarsia and round facies and subcutaneous bone formation.

Type Ib and Ic have normal Gs-alpha protein but in type Ic the patients have resistance to multiple hormones. Type Ic also has phenotype of Albright's hereditary osteodystrophy and often present with short stature. Type Ia and Ic have autosomal dominant mode of inheritance. Type Ib is mostly sporadic but familial cases have been reported. Type Ib has a defective kidney response to PTH.

In type II, the defect lies downstream after the generation of cyclic AMP as the levels increase normally but it fails to raise the level of serum calcium or urinary phosphate secretion. These patients present with a typical picture suggesting vitamin D deficiency but in vitamin D deficiency the parameters become normal after supplementation with it which does not happen in these cases.

Low PTH causes of hypocalcemia
- Genetic disorders
- Abnormal development of parathyroid gland
- Abnormal synthesis of PTH
- Activating mutations of the calcium-sensing receptor

Postsurgical
- Due to inadvertent removal during thyroidectomy
- Parathyroidectomy
- Radical neck dissection

Autoimmune
- Part of autoimmune polyglandular syndrome
- Isolated hypoparathyroidism due to activating antibodies to calcium-sensing receptor

Parathyroid gland infiltration
- Granulomatous
- Iron overload
- Metastasis
- Radiation-induced damage to parathyroid (can happen after radioiodine ablation of thyroid gland also)
- Hungry bone syndrome (post-parathyroidectomy)
- HIV infection

High PTH causes of hypocalcemia

Vitamin D deficiency or resistance

Parathyroid hormone resistance
- Pseudohypoparathyroidism
- Hypomagnesemia
- Renal failure

Loss of calcium from circulation
- Hyperphosphatemia
- Tumor lysis syndrome
- Acute pancreatitis
- Sepsis or acute severe illness
- Osteoblastic metastasis
- Acute respiratory alkalosis

Q. 8 What is the diagnostic approach for a case of hypocalcemia?

Ans. The first step in the diagnosis is to confirm that true hypocalcemia is present. An acute transient hypocalcemia can be a manifestation of a variety of severe, acute illnesses. Chronic hypocalcemia, however, can usually be ascribed to a few disorders associated with absent or ineffective PTH. Important clinical criteria include the duration of the illness, signs or symptoms of associated disorders, and the presence of features that suggest a hereditary abnormality. A nutritional history can be helpful in recognizing a low intake of vitamin D and calcium in the diet and a history of excessive alcohol intake may suggest magnesium deficiency (Flowchart 15.1).

FLOWCHART 15.1 Diagnostic approach to a patient with hypocalcemia

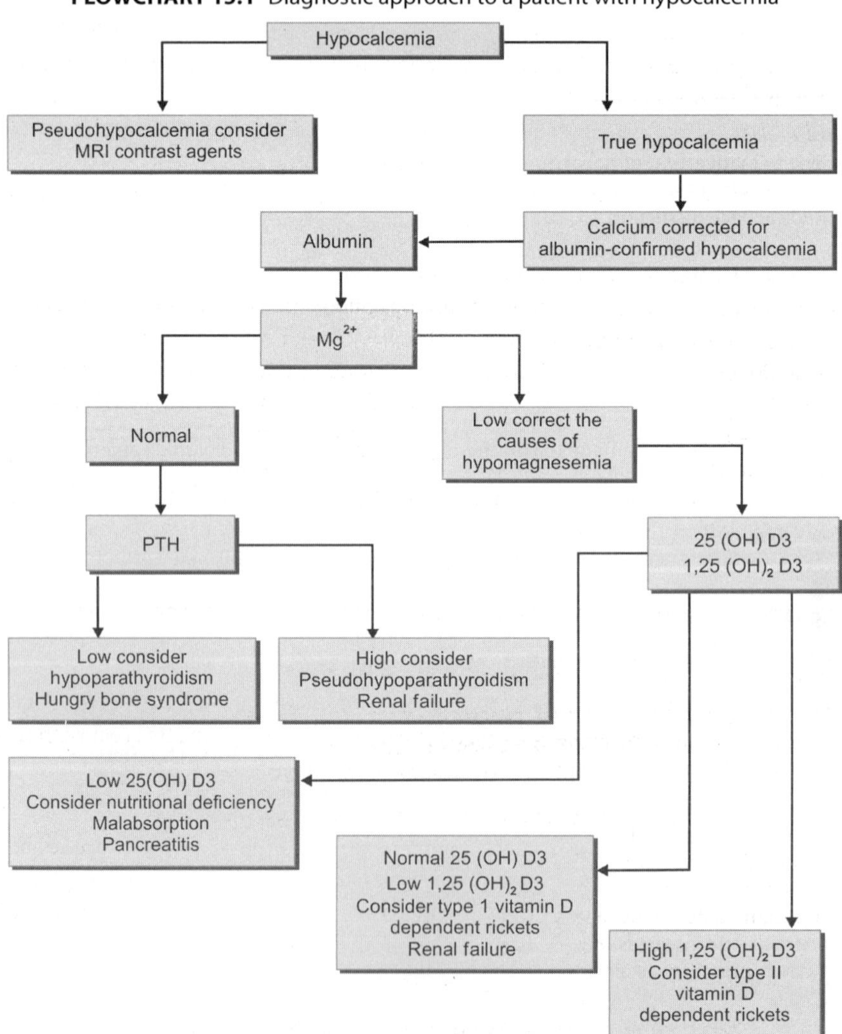

Q. 9 How should a case of hypocalcemia be managed in the emergency room?

Ans. Management comprises of:

- Suspecting that patient has hypocalcemia
- Measurement and correct interpretation of serum calcium levels
- Initiating emergency calcium replacement and this can be done, without waiting for the serum calcium levels
- A further detailed analysis to find a cause for hypocalcemia in the patient so as to avoid recurrences of similar episodes.

Q. 10 What is the normal function of the ionized calcium?

Ans. Ionized calcium is the necessary plasma fraction for normal physiologic processes. In the neuromuscular system, ionized calcium facilitates nerve conduction, muscle contraction, and muscle relaxation.

Q. 11 What is the most common cause of total serum calcium low in the body with ionized calcium levels being normal and how to calculate corrected calcium value?

Ans. The most common cause is low albumin level because of any condition like cirrhosis, nephropathy, malnutrition, burns, chronic illness, and sepsis.

To correct for hypoalbuminemia, add 0.8 mg/dL to the total serum calcium for each 1.0 g/dL decrease in albumin below 4.0 g/dL.

Q. 12 Is the measurement of magnesium important in this patient?

Ans. Yes ideally, serum magnesium levels should also be measured in each patient having these symptoms. Because sustained correction of hypocalcemia cannot be achieved by administration of calcium alone in patients of hypomagnesemia; but administration of magnesium corrects the hypocalcemia in such patients.

Yes, some patients with magnesium-responsive hypocalcemia have normal serum magnesium concentrations. These patients are presumed to have tissue magnesium deficiency. Thus, magnesium supplementation may be indicated in patients with unexplained hypocalcemia who are at risk for hypomagnesemia, such as patients with chronic malabsorption or alcoholism.

Hypomagnesemia should always be looked for in patients with hypocalcemia.

Q. 13 How magnesium deficiency causes hypocalcemia?

Ans. Magnesium deficiency causes hypocalcemia by producing PTH resistance and this happens when serum magnesium falls below 0.8 mg/dL and with more severe hypomagnesemia PTH secretion is also affected.

Q. 14 How can acid-base imbalance precipitate hypocalcemia?

Ans. Alkalosis (e.g. induced by hyperventilation), hypokalemia, epinephrine (e.g. due to emotional stress), and hypomagnesemia aggravate symptoms of hypocalcemia; whereas acidosis diminishes symptoms, as seen in patients with chronic renal failure who often tolerate marked hypocalcemia without symptoms.

Start calcium replacement without waiting for the results when in doubt.

Q. 15 What are the clinical manifestations of hypocalcemia?

Ans. The clinical symptoms and signs include signs of neuromuscular irritability such as Chvostek's sign, Trousseau's sign, Erb's sign, paraesthesias in circumoral and acral areas (fingers and toes), muscle stiffness, myalgias and laryngeal spasms may happen in severe cases the neuropsychiatric symptoms include seizures which can be of any type but commonly grand mal seizure, dementia in adults, mental retardation in children, emotional problems such as anxiety, depression, irritability and psychosis, extrapyramidal symptoms such as parkinsonian-like features, calcification of the basal ganglia may happen in long-standing disease and papilledema because of raised intracranial tension.

Q. 16 Do they have any cardiovascular manifestations?

Ans. The cardiovascular manifestations include prolongation of the QT interval, congestive heart failure, hypotension and arrhythmias.

Q. 17 Can they have autonomic symptoms?

Ans. Yes, it can be in the form of biliary colic, diaphoresis and bronchospasm.

Q. 18 What other symptoms can be present?

Ans. This includes cataract, dry and coarse skin, dermatitis, hyperpigmentation and eczema, steatorrhea and gastric achlorhydria.

Q. 19 What is Erb's sign?

Ans. This was considered to be the most reliable proof of tetany in the earlier times before the biochemical tests were available, and it include increased excitability of the peripheral nerves to the galvanic current.

Q. 20 Measurement and correct interpretation of serum calcium levels.

Ans. Total calcium in serum (8.7–10.2 mg/dL) includes—free ions, ions bound to albumin, and to a small extent, diffusible complexes. The concentration of free calcium ions, averaging 4.8 mg/dL, influences many cellular functions and is subjected to tight hormonal control, especially through PTH.

In a patient with hypocalcemia, the serum albumin is essential to the diagnosis of true hypocalcemia which involves a reduction in ionized serum calcium, or to the diagnosis of "factitious" hypocalcemia, meaning decreased total, but not ionized calcium.

It is thus more useful to measure serum free calcium ion levels using calcium electrodes. If ionized calcium cannot be measured, an approximation can be used to estimate the protein-bound and ionized fractions.

A formula that estimates the amount of corrected calcium is:

Corrected calcium = [0.8 × (4 – serum albumin)] + serum calcium.

Q. 21 What is the formula to measure serum calcium in sick patients?

Ans. However, no formula has proved accurate for assessment of serum calcium concentration in acutely ill patients. Critically-ill patients may have transient hypocalcemia with severe sepsis, burns, acute renal failure, extensive transfusions with citrated blood, and infusion of large amounts of albumin. Drugs used in critical care settings such as heparin, protamine, and glucagon may also induce a transient hypocalcemia. In most of the cases, the major cause for hypocalcemia is hypoalbuminemia. Other causes of hypocalcemia in the critically ill patient include alkalosis (alkalosis increases calcium binding to proteins), hypomagnesemia, elevated circulating free fatty acids, and lipid infusions.

Ionized calcium can be helpful when the diagnosis is considered in the setting of acute illness or severe hypoalbuminemia.

Q. 22 How is calcium replacement done in emergency in patient with hypocalcemia?

Ans. Patients with acute symptomatic hypocalcemia (serum calcium usually below 7.0 mg/dL, and ionized calcium usually below 3.2 mg/dL) should be treated promptly with IV calcium. Calcium gluconate is preferred option over calcium chloride because it causes less tissue necrosis, if extravasated. The first 100–200 mg of elemental calcium (1–2 ampoules of 10% calcium gluconate [93 mg/10 mL ampoule]) should be given over 10–20 minutes. Calcium for infusion should be diluted in 50–100 mL of saline or 5% dextrose solution to avoid vein irritation. Faster administration may result in cardiac dysfunction, even arrest. This should be followed by slow calcium infusion at 0.5–2 mg/kg/hr which can be done by adding 10 ampoules of calcium gluconate in 500 mL of 5% dextrose. Calcium infusion should be continued until the patient is receiving effective doses of oral calcium (1–3 g of elemental calcium daily) and vitamin D and is maintaining normal calcium levels. The infusion solution should not contain bicarbonate or phosphate because these can form insoluble calcium salts. If bicarbonate or phosphate administration is necessary, a separate IV line should be used.

Serum calcium should be measured every 4–6 hours to maintain serum calcium levels at 8–9 mg/dL. Patients with cardiac arrhythmias or patients on digoxin therapy need continuous ECG monitoring during calcium replacement because calcium potentiates digitalis toxicity.

Coexisting hypomagnesemia (serum Mg levels <1.8 mg/dL) should be considered in every patient, and if present or if the magnesium status is unknown, magnesium should be supplemented. Great care should be taken in patients with impaired renal function because they cannot excrete excess magnesium. Magnesium is given in an infusion and initiated with 2 g magnesium sulfate over 10–15 minutes followed by 1 g/hr.

The cause of hypocalcemia in this patient is pseudohypoparathyroidism. The above mentioned patient is started on calcium infusion and also started on oral calcium supplementation and active vitamin D. She recovers with treatment and is continued on calcium and active vitamin D.

CASE 2

A 41-year-old female with a history of Graves' disease is admitted to our hospital for further evaluation and treatment of hypocalcemia. She gives a history of receiving radioactive iodine supplementation for the treatment of her Graves' disease about 6 years back, when she received dose of 10 millicurie and after 3 months of the ablation patient became hypothyroid and was started on levothyroxine supplementation in a dose of 125 µg per day and henceforth she has been maintaining a normal calcium level. She has no family history of bone and mineral metabolism disorders. She was diagnosed as severe hypocalcemia 1 week back (serum corrected calcium level, 6.7 mg/dL) and referred to our hospital. On admission, her blood pressure is 100/76 mm Hg, and her pulse rate is 68 beats/minute with regular rhythm. Her thyroid gland is barely palpable. Her heart and breathing sounds are clear. Trousseau and Chvostek signs are positive. Chest X-ray is normal. Electrocardiogram shows a prolonged QTc interval (0.49 msec).

Q. 1 What investigations are needed in this case?

Ans. The blood chemistry shows low serum corrected calcium level (6.3 mg/dL) and fasting serum phosphate level is 6.5 mg/dL (range 2.5 mg/dL to 4.5 mg/dL), normal magnesium level (2.4 mg/dL), and normal alkaline phosphatase level (160 U/L). There is no renal and liver dysfunction. Endocrine examinations shows that serum 25(OH)D level is markedly decreased (<5 ng/mL), and intact PTH (iPTH) and 1,25$(OH)_2$D levels are low (5 pg/mL and 23 pg/mL). Thyroid function is in normal range (*See* Flowchart 15.1).

Lab tests-initial
- Serum calcium
- Serum phosphorus
- Serum magnesium
- Serum albumin
- Serum alkaline phosphatase
- 25 (OH) D
- 1,25$(OH)_2$D
- Intact PTH
- Serum creatinine

The blood chemistry shows low serum corrected calcium level (6.3 mg/dL) and fasting serum phosphate level is 6.5 mg/dL (normal range 2.5–4.5 mg/dL), normal magnesium level (2.4 mg/dL), and normal alkaline phosphatase level (160 U/L). There is no evidence of renal and liver dysfunction. Endocrine examinations shows that serum 25(OH)D level are markedly decreased (<5 ng/mL), and intact PTH (iPTH) and 1,25$(OH)_2$D levels are low (5 pg/mL and 23 pg/mL). Thyroid function is in normal range.

Q. 2 What is the cause of low serum calcium in this lady's case?

Ans. From her clinical course and laboratory findings, we diagnose that her numbness in hands and lip is due to hypocalcemia probably caused by hypoparathyroidism secondary to the radioactive iodine ablation and has been exacerbated by concurrent vitamin D deficiency. The explanation is that if it would have only be contributed by vitamin D deficiency her PTH should have been high and her phosphorus should have been normal or below normal but not high.

Q. 3 What is the possible reason for low serum calcium after radioiodine ablation?

Ans. Radioactive iodine ablation can damage parathyroid tissue and cause hypocalcemia if administered in large doses since β particles emitted by ^{131}I can penetrate up to 2.5 mm into surrounding tissues. Intrathyroidal parathyroid glands, present in about 4% of adults, may be at increased risk for destruction.

Q. 4 What is the cause of low phosphorus in a patient with PTH deficiency or resistance due to any cause?

Ans. The elevated serum phosphate concentration in patients with either disorder is due to loss of the stimulatory effect of PTH on urinary phosphate excretion and is therefore associated with an inappropriately low fractional excretion of phosphate.

Q. 5 What is the treatment for this lady?

Ans. The lady has to be treated with calcium and vitamin D because concurrent deficiency of vitamin D in this lady has precipitated hypocalcemia.

She is started on oral calcium carbonate supplements of 3 g per day after food in divided doses with 1,25-dihydroxy vitamin D (activated form of vitamin D) in a dose of 1.5 mg per day in 3 divided dosages. Her calcium levels have increased to 8.5 mg/dL after 2 days of treatment and she is continued on this treatment and discharged from the hospital and is called after 2 weeks. She continues to have normal calcium levels.

Q. 6 Do we routinely need to monitor all patients postradioiodine ablation for hypocalcemia?

Ans. No, hypocalcemia after radioiodine ablation is rare and no recommendation exists for routine screening for hypocalcemia postradioiodine ablation.

SUGGESTED READING

1. Antakia R, Edafe O, Uttley L, Balasubramanian SP. Effectiveness of preventative and other surgical measures on hypocalcemia following bilateralthyroid surgery: a systematic review and meta-analysis. Thyroid. 2015;25(1):95-106.
2. Barak S, Baker HWG. In: De Groot LJ, Beck-Peccoz P, Chrousos G, Dungan K, Grossman A,Hershman JM, Koch C, McLachlan R, New M, Rebar R, Singer F, Vinik A, Weickert MO (Eds). Endotext [Internet]. South Dartmouth (MA): MDText.com, Inc.; 2000-. Available from *http://www.ncbi.nlm.nih.gov/books/NBK279022/PubMed PMID: 25905251.*
3. Cole DEC, Hendy GN, Bastepe M. Hypoparathyroidism and Pseudohypoparathyroidism. 2011 Aug 1. In: De Groot LJ, Beck-Peccoz P, Chrousos G, Dungan K, Grossman A, Hershman JM, Koch C, McLachlan R, New M, Rebar R, Singer F,Vinik A, Weickert MO (Eds). Endotext [Internet]. South Dartmouth (MA):MDText.com, Inc.; 2000. Available from *http://www.ncbi.nlm.nih.gov/books/NBK279165/PubMed PMID: 25905388.* Schafer AL, Fitzpatrick LA, Shoback DM. Hypocalcemia: Diagnosis and Treatment.
4. Fallah-Rad N, Morton AR. Managing hypercalcaemia and hypocalcaemia in cancer patients. Curr Opin Support Palliat Care. 2013;7(3):265-71.

5. Fong J, Khan A. Hypocalcemia: updates in diagnosis and management for primary care. Can Fam Physician. 2012;58(2):158-62. Review.
6. Hoorn EJ, Zietse R. Disorders of calcium and magnesium balance: a physiology-based approach. Pediatr Nephrol. 2013;28(8):1195-206. doi:10.1007/s00467-012-2350-2. Epub 2012 Nov 10. Review.
7. Seo ST, Chang JW, Jin J, Lim YC, Rha KS, Koo BS. Transient and permanent hypocalcemia after total thyroidectomy: early predictive factors and long-term follow-up results. Surgery. 2015 Jul 2. pii: S0039-6060(15)00444-4.
8. Shaw NJ. A practical approach to hypocalcaemia in children. Endocr Dev. 2015;28: 84-100. doi: 10.1159/000380997. Epub 2015 Jun 12.

CHAPTER

16

Approach to Hypercalcemia

Madhukar Mittal, Neelam Yadav

CASE 1

A 54-year-old female presents with drowsiness to the emergency.

Her BP is 140/90 mm of Hg with pulse after rate 100/minute.

Her investigations reveals serum creatinine 2.4 mg/dL, Na 140 mEq/L, K 4.3 mEq/L. Complete blood count (CBC) and liver function test (LFT) is normal. CT scan head is normal.

Her past evaluation reveals a cervical lymph node fine needle aspiration cytology (FNAC) suggestive of granulomatous inflammation.

Her bone marrow examination is suggestive of non-Hodgkin's lymphoma.

Q. 1 What history and examination would you like to assess?

Ans. History of diabetes or diabetic medication intake.

Neurological examination for signs of meningeal irritation or focal neurological deficit.

Case: Her serum calcium report is 16 mg/dL.

Q. 2 What are the manifestations of hypercalcemia?

Ans.

- Gastrointestinal (GI)—anorexia, nausea, vomiting, gastroesophageal-reflux disease (GERD), peptic ulcer, acute pancreatitis.
- Renal—polyuria (decreased urinary concentrating ability), nephrocalcinosis, nephrolithiasis.
- Cardiovascular system (CVS)—hypertension, bradycardia, shortened QT interval on ECG.
- Central nervous system (CNS)—weakness, fatigue, lassitude, depression, confusion, stupor, coma.

Q. 3 What investigations would you order in a case of hypercalcemia?

Ans. The recommended investigations are:

- Serum calcium total and ionized
- Serum albumin

- Serum phosphorus
- 25(OH)D
- Serum iPTH.

Q. 4 What constitutes hypercalcemia?

Ans. Serum calcium levels ≥10.5 mg/dL constitutes hypercalcemia. The normal serum calcium (Ca) levels are maintained by a coordinated interaction between 4 important organ-systems/glands:

I—Parathyroid gland
II—Kidneys
III—Intestine
IV—Bone.

Q. 5 What is the role of various organs in calcium metabolism?

Ans.

Organ-systems/gland	Role
Parathyroid gland	Parathyroid hormone (PTH) secretion
Kidneys	1,25$(OH)_2$D formation
Intestine	Calcium absorption
Bone	Store of calcium

The blood levels of calcium are maintained within the normal range by interplay of the above factors.

Q. 6 What are the functions of calcium in the body?

Ans.

- Structural component of bone and teeth (over 99% of the 1–2 kg of Ca present in adult human body resides in the skeleton)
- Participates in enzymatic functions
  - Muscular contraction
  - Blood coagulation
  - Digestive enzymes
- Second messenger for some hormonal actions
- Release of neurotransmitters, e.g. noradrenaline, acetylcholine at NM junction.

Q. 7 How is calcium absorbed in the body?

Ans. *Gastrointestinal absorption of calcium*

Calcium is absorbed in the small intestine predominantly in the duodenum and jejunum. The gastrointestinal (GI) absorption of calcium is by various means:

- Passive (paracellular)—5%
- Active (transcellular)—20–70%

It is controlled by 1,25$(OH)_2$D. 1,25$(OH)_2$D induces calbindin which promotes active transport of calcium across the intestine. The GI absorption requires the presence of gastric acid. So, whenever calcium carbonate tablets are prescribed, they are advised to be taken with meals. In achlorhydric subjects, it is preferable to use calcium citrate tablets instead.

Renal absorption of calcium

PCT (65%)	Passive
cTAL (20%)	Paracellular
	Inhibits by ↑ serum Ca/Mg via the CaSR directly
DCT (10%)	Transcellular
	Thiazides lower urinary Ca excretion
	Loop diuretics/saline infusion ↓ DCT Ca reabsorption

Increased calcium reabsorption is promoted by PTH and 1,25$(OH)_2$D.

Patient's serum phosphorus is 3.6 mg/dL. 25(OH)D level is 36 ng/mL and serum PTH is 50 pg/mL.

She is immediately started on IV fluids (Normal saline) with furosemide 20 mg 8 hourly. Calcitonin SC is also given for 2 days. Zoledronate intravenous infusion 5 mg single dose is also given. Serum calcium levels are monitored daily—subsequent values are 14 mg/dL, 11.5 mg/dL, 10.6 mg/dL, 8.8 mg/dL. Serum creatinine value comes down to 1.0 mg/dL.

Q. 8 How do we treat a case of hypercalcemia?

Ans.

- Hydration with saline
  NS at 300–500 mL/hour
  Up to 3–4 L in first 24 hours
- Forced diuresis — NS at 100–200 mL/hour
  + furosemide IV 20–40 mg BD/QID
  S/E — Potassium and Mg depletion
  Renal Ca calculi
  Volume overload and pulmonary edema
- Bisphosphonates
  Onset of action over 1–2 days
  Inhibits osteoclast action by complex mechanisms

2nd generation	Pamidronate	30–90 mg in 500 mL NS/5%D over 4 hours
3rd generation	Zoledronate	4–5 mg IV infusion over 30 min
	S/E of infusion	Fever in 20%
		↓ Ca, P, Mg

- Calcitonin—2–8 U/kg SC/IM/IV every 6–12 hour
  Onset of action within hours
  Tachyphylaxis after 24 hours of use
  Safe in renal failure
  Mechanism of action—blocks bone resorption via receptors on osteoclasts
  Inhibits renal tubular Ca reabsorption → ↑ urinary Ca excretion

Treatment approach

Mild hypercalcemia → 1

Severe hypercalcemia → 2 + 3 + 4

Intermediate hypercalcemia → 1 + 2/3/4.......

Q. 9 What are the other drugs for treating hypercalcemia?

Ans.

- *Glucocorticoids*

  Use in → Malignancy related local osteolytic hypercalcemia
  Vitamin D/A intoxication
  Sarcoidosis

  Prednisolone 20–50 mg BD (40–100 mg/day)
- *Oral phosphate*

  For chronic management in patients with hypophosphatemia
  1–1.5 g/day of phosphorus in divided doses
  IV phosphate in severe hypercalcemia + cardiac/renal failure
  Phosphate dose >1500 mg over 6–8 hours
  S/E ectopic calcification, renal damage, fatal hypocalcemia
- *Dialysis:* Useful in renal failure
- Obsolete
  - Plicamycin (Mithramycin) 25 μg/kg IV
    S/E—N, hepatotoxicity, proteinuria, thrombocytopenia
  - Gallium nitrate.

Review of bone marrow slides showed no evidence of NHL. Cervical lymph node biopsy was done which revealed tuberculous lymphadenopathy.

Q. 10 What is the role of vitamin D in bone metabolism?

Ans. 1,25$(OH)_2$D → Stimulates 24α-hydroxylase
Inhibits 1α-hydroxylase

1α-hydroxylase is present in:

- Proximal tubular cells of kidney
- Epidermal keratinocytes
- Trophoblastic layer of placenta
- Granulomas of sarcoidosis, TB, berylliosis
- Site for vitamin D receptors include intestine, pancreas, bone, skeletal muscle, kidney, vascular smooth muscle, skin (epidermal keratinocytes), lymphocytes. Not in liver.

Q. 11 What is the role of PTH?

Ans. Parathyroid hormone (PTH) is an 84-amino acid single chain peptide. The amino acid portion PTH (1-34) is critical for its biologic action. It is secreted as preproparathyroid hormone (115 aa) → Proparathyroid hormone (90 aa) (aa, amino acid).

Actions of PTH

PTH Increases rate of dissolution of bone mineral
Renal action: ↑ reabsorption of Ca (distal tubule)
Inhibition of phosphate transport (proximal tubule)
Stimulation of 25(OH)D 1α-hydroxylase
Inhibits 24-hydroxylase

Receptors for PTH PTH1R Responds to PTH and PTHrP
PTH2R Responds to PTH only

PTH-related peptide (PTHrP) is secreted by some squamous cell tumors. It is also secreted by mammary tissue (secreted into milk).

Decreased PTH release and synthesis occurs by:

- Calcium (ionized form) acting through CaSR (hypercalcemia)
- $1,25(OH)_2D$
- Hypermagnesemia
- Severe hypomagnesemia.

Q. 12 How to measure serum calcium?

Ans.

	mg/dL	*mmol/L*	*Peak*	*Nadir*
Total calcium	9.0–10.4	2.2–2.6	1:00 pm	10:00 am
Ionized calcium	4.5–5.2	1.1–1.3	3:00 am	6–8 pm

Serum calcium should be measured in fasting state. Acidosis decreases the association of calcium with protein. Correction of serum calcium is 0.8 times the deficit in serum albumin in g/dL or 0.5 times the deficit in serum globulin in g/dL.

Percentage protein bound calcium = [0.8 × albumin (g/L)] + [0.2 × globulin (g/L)] + 3

Corrected calcium level (mg%) = serum calcium (mg%) + [4 – serum albumin (g%) × 0.8]

Q. 13 What is the grading of hypercalcemia?

Ans.

Mild	10.5–12.0 mg/dL	
Intermediate	12.0–15.0 mg/dL	Calcification in kidneys, skin, vessels Renal insufficiency
Severe	>15.0–18.0 mg/dL	Frequent with parathyroid CA

$1,25(OH)_2D$ values were high normal and PTHrP values were awaited. She was started on antituberculous treatment.

Serum calcium values on follow-up were 8.0 mg/dL and 8.8 mg/dL.

Q. 14 What is the most probable cause of hypercalcemia in this patient?

a. Primary hyperparathyroidism
b. Non-Hodgkin's lymphoma
c. Tuberculosis
d. Acute renal failure

Ans. Tuberculosis

Q. 15 What are the causes of hypercalcemia?

Ans.

- Primary hyperparathyroidism
  - Adenoma — Hereditary causes – HRPT2(HPT-JT)
  - Hyperplasia — Hereditary causes – MEN1, MEN2A, HRPT1
- Malignancy (2nd MC cause)
  - Humoral hypercalcemia of malignancy (PTHrP) Ca lung, kidney, head and neck, urogenital tract
  - Osteolytic bone metastases

  - Hematological malignancies—lymphoma, leukemia, multiple myeloma (↑ESR, Normal SALP)
  - Both breast Ca, HTLV-1 induced adult T-cell leukemia
  - Ectopic tumor produced PTH
- **R**eset parathyroid CaSR
  - Familial hypocalciuric hypercalcemia
  - Lithium
- **V**itamin D related
  - Vitamin D intoxication
  - ↑1,25$(OH)_2$D Granulomatous disease—sarcoidosis, TB, fungal infections
  - Williams syndrome (idiopathic hypercalcemia of infancy)
- **A**ssociated with high bone turnover
  - Immobilization
  - Endocrine hyperthyroidism, acromegaly, pheochromocytoma
- **A**ssociated with renal failure
  - Aluminum (Al) intoxication
  - Milk alkali syndrome
  - Severe secondary hyperparathyroidism
- **Others**
  - Exogenous PTH therapy
  - Jansen's disease.

Q. 16 What is vitamin D intoxication and how does it present?

Ans. It is due to excessive biologic actions of elevated levels of 25(OH)D. Diagnosis is by 25(OH)D levels >100 ng/mL. It is increasingly been seen with unregulated overuse of vitamin D in therapeutic doses without measuring blood levels. 1,25$(OH)_2$D levels may not be elevated (because they are tightly regulated). Treatment is to stop intake of vitamin D. Maintaining adequate hydration and Hydrocortisone 100 mg/day may be helpful. Hypercalcemia may persist for weeks as vitamin D stores in fat may be substantial.

Q. 17 Can sarcoidosis lead to hypercalcemia?

Ans. Hypercalcemia in sarcoidosis occurs due to excess unregulated 1,25$(OH)_2$D synthesized in macrophages in granulomas. There is a positive correlation between 25(OH)D levels (reflecting vitamin D intake) and the circulating concentration of 1,25$(OH)_2$D. This is normally not the case as there is no increase in 1,25$(OH)_2$D with increasing 25(OH)D levels due to multiple feedback controls on renal 1α-hydroxylase. These controls are lost in granulomatous diseases like sarcoidosis.

↑ 1,25$(OH)_2$D , ↓ PTH → hypercalciuria

Treatment is to ↓ intake of vitamin D, avoid excessive sunlight exposure, and hydrocortisone. Hypercalcemia of sarcoidosis is usually associated with disseminated disease. Almost all have abnormal chest X-ray (CXR). Sarcoidosis is unlikely as a cause of hypercalcemia, if CXR is normal. Hypergammaglobulinemia is a clue to the disease.

William's Syndrome

It is an autosomal dominant disorder characterized by Elfin facies, mental retardation, supravalvular aortic stenosis. The hypercalcemia is due to abnormal sensitivity to vitamin D. Increased levels of 1,25$(OH)_2$D are seen.

Vitamin A Intoxication

This is an uncommon cause for hypercalcemia and is usually due to dietary faddism. It is presumed to be due to increased bone resorption. Periosteal calcifications, especially in hands may be seen. Diagnosis is by elevated serum vitamin A levels. Treatment includes stopping vitamin A intake and hydrocortisone.

Thiazides

Thiazide diuretics like hydrochlorothiazide induce hypocalciuria due to increased proximal tubular resorption of Na and Ca in response to sodium depletion. They can cause hypercalcemia in patients with high rates of bone turnover which is usually mild.

Immobilization

Hypercalcemia is seen with prolonged immobilization, especially after spinal cord injury and paraplegia or quadriplegia. This is more common in children or adolescents.

Hyperthyroidism

Hypercalciuria is more common than hypercalcemia. Mild hypercalcemia occurs in around 20% of patients.

Aluminum Intoxication

This is nowadays no longer seen. It used to occur in patients on chronic hemodialysis with aluminum in the dialysis regimen. Patients may present with acute dementia, unresponsive and severe osteomalacia with bone pain, multiple fractures, especially of ribs and pelvis and proximal myopathy. When these patients on chronic hemodialysis are treated with vitamin D, hypercalcemia results. Aluminum is present at the site of osteoid mineralization but osteoblastic activity is minimal. The calcium incorporation into the skeleton is impaired in these individuals. Treatment is to avoid aluminum excess in the dialysis regimen and deferoxamine.

Milk Alkali Syndrome

This is a triad of hypercalcemia, metabolic alkalosis and renal insufficiency. The chronic form of the disease associated with irreversible renal damage is known as Burnett syndrome. It results due to excessive ingestion of Calcium via absorbable antacids (e.g. milk, $CaCO_3$). Investigations reveal ↑HCO_3, ↑Serum creatinine, and decreased chloride.

Q. 18 How do we differentiate malignancy-related hypercalcemia?

Ans.

What is same as in primary hyperparathyroidism?
↑ Urinary phosphate clearance
Hypophosphatemia
↑ Urinary nephrogenous cAMP excretion

What is different from primary hyperparathyroidism?
↓ PTH (by double antibody technique)
↑ Renal calcium clearance
↓/N levels of ↑ $1,25(OH)_2D$
Other paraneoplastic syndromes
Elevated levels of PTHrP may be detected

Investigations

Radiology Osteolytic metastases may be seen on X-ray
Tc-labeled bisphosphonate bone scan may detect metastases
BM biopsy in patients with hematological abnormality
Chest X-ray
CT abdomen

Treatment of hypercalcemia is first directed to control of tumor. Reduction of tumor mass usually controls hypercalcemia.

Q. 19 What is familial hypocalciuric hypercalcemia (FHH)?

Ans. This is an autosomal dominant but is a cause for asymptomatic hypercalcemia. No treatment is usually required except in case of neonatal severe hypercalcemia due to homozygous or compound heterozygote state where total parathyroidectomy is mandatory. This condition is due to loss of function mutations in CaSR which results in abnormal sensing of blood calcium and increased secretion of PTH. There is an increased renal reabsorption of calcium.

Q. 20 What is different in FHH from primary hyperparathyroidism?

Ans. Familial hypocalciuric hyprcalcemia (FHH) is often detectable in affected members of the kindred in the first decade of life.

PTH values are usually lower for the same degree of calcium elevation than in patients with primary hyperparathyroidism.

Renal calcium reabsorption is >99% (↓ 24 hour urinary Ca).

Hypocalciuria persists even after parathyroid surgery, i.e. hypocalciuria is not PTH dependent.

Q. 21 What is Jansen disease?

Ans. This is an autosomal dominant condition resulting from constitutive receptor functioning. It occurs due to mutations in PTH1R. ↑Ca, ↓Phosphate, ↓PTH is seen.

Short-limbed dwarfism occurs due to abnormal regulation of bone growth plate.

Multiple cystic resorptive areas in bone occur, similar to those seen in severe primary hyperparathyroidism.

CASE 2

A young female of 24 years, presents with bony pains and difficulty in walking for 2 years. Her plain radiographs show fractures of right shaft of tibia and fibula and diffuse osteopenia. Screw and plating was seen at right femur for which patient gives a past history of fracture due to trivial trauma 3 years back. Her biochemical parameters reveal serum Ca 13.4 mg/dL, serum phosphorus 1.4 mg/dL, serum creatinine 1.2 mg/dL. Hb is 11.0 g%. 25(OH)D value is 45 ng/dL and her PTH is 108 pg/mL. USG abdomen shows left renal calculus. BMD shows severe osteoporosis.

Her past history reveals being treated for 6 months for pulmonary tuberculosis 4 years back. Her mother expired from non-Hodgkin's lymphoma 12 years back.

Q. 1 What is her diagnosis?

a. Primary hyperparathyroidism
b. Non-Hodgkin's lymphoma
c. Tuberculosis
d. Acute renal failure

Ans. Primary hyperparathyroidism

Q. 2 How does primary hyperparathyroidism present?

Ans. Central nervous system (CNS)—fatigue, depression, psychosis
Neuromusculars—myopathy, pseudogout
GIT—constipation, peptic ulcer, GERD, pancreatitis
Renal—polyuria, renal stones (Ca oxalate, Ca phosphate), nephrocalcinosis
CVS—hypertension, ↓ QT interval, arrhythmias, vascular calcification
Skeletal
- Osteitis fibrosa cystica
- ↑ osteoclasts in Howship's lacunae
- Brown tumors (hemorrhagic cystic lesions)
- Subperiosteal resorption
- ↓ cortical bone density (cancellous bone preserved, especially in spine)
- Fractures
- ?Marrow fibrosis

Asymptomatic in >50%

Q. 3 How would you investigate a case of primary hyperparathyroidism on follow-up?

Ans. Serums calcium Biannually
Serum creatinine Annually
Bone mineral density Annually
Initially 24 hour urinary Ca
Creatinine clearance
Abdominal X-ray + USG

Q. 4 What are the indications for surgery in primary hyperparathyroidism?

Ans. Serum calcium >1.0 mg/dL above upper limit of normal
24 hours urinary Ca >400 mg/day
Creatinine clearance ↓ by 30%
Age <50 year
Complications of primary hyperparathyroidism (PHPT) including:

- Nephrocalcinosis
- Osteoporosis (T-score <2.5 SD at the lumbar spine, hip, or wrist)
- Severe psychoneurologic disorder

Who cannot participate in appropriate follow-up.

Q. 5 What is postoperative hypocalcemia?

Ans. Decline in serum Ca occurs within 24 hours of successful surgery; lasts for 3–5 days
Once hypocalcemia occurs, it signifies successful surgery
- Give High Ca intake, Oral Ca supplements

If serum calcium persistently <8 mg/dL + Phosphate level rises → consider that surgery has caused hypoparathyroidism
With unexpected hypocalcemia → consider coexistent hypomagnesemia
Parenteral Ca when hypocalcemia is symptomatic : IV Ca 1–2 mg/kg/hour
If asymptomatic → No treatment required

Q. 6 What are the causes of hypercalciuria?

Ans.

- Causes of hypercalcemia except FHH, thiazides, Addison's disease
- Idiopathic hypercalciuria
- Renal tubular acidosis (RTA) I and II
- Bartter syndrome

Q. 7 What are the causes of nephrolithiasis and nephrocalcinosis?

Ans.

- Causes of hypercalciuria
  - Idiopathic hypercalciuria
  - Renal tubular acidosis (RTA) I and II
  - Bartter syndrome
  - Causes of hypercalcemia except familial hypocalciuric hypercalcemia (FHH), thiazides, Addison's disease
- Causes of hyperoxaluria
- Medullary sponge kidney
- Renal papillary necrosis

APPROACH TO HYPERCALCEMIA

Serum Ca	*Serum PO_4*	*Serum PTH*		*DDx*	
↑	↓	↑	→	1° hyperparathyroidism FHH Lithium	
↑	↓	↓	→	Malignancy Jansen's disease	
↑	↑	↓	→	Hypervitaminosis D Sarcoidosis, etc. William's syndrome	↑ 25(OH)D ↑ 1,25$(OH)_2$D
N	N	N	→	Osteoporosis Osteogenesis imperfecta Hypercalcitoninemia (MTC) Paget disease	 ↑ SALP

Abbreviation: SALP, serum alkaline phosphatase

CALCIUM SALTS

Calcium salt	*% elemental Ca*	*Calcium content (per g)*	*Ca salt per ampoule*
Ca carbonate	40	400 mg	1 g/5 mL
Ca citrate	21	211 mg	
Tricalcium phosphate	39	390	
Ca lactate	13	130	
Ca glubionate	7	64	1.8 g/5 mL
Ca gluconate	9	93	1 g/10 mL
Ca chloride (IV)	36	360	1 g/10 mL

- Most common cause of hypercalcemia is primary hyperparathyroidism.
- Most common cause of hypercalcemia in a hospitalized patient is secondary to malignancy.

SUGGESTED READING

1. Bandeira L, Bilezikian J. Primary Hyperparathyroidism. F1000Research. 2016;5:F1000 Faculty Rev-1.
2. Cusano NE, Silverberg SJ, Bilezikian JP. Normocalcemic Primary Hyperparathyroidism. Journal of Clinical Densitometry: the Official Journal of the International Society for Clinical Densitometry. 2013;16(1):33-9.
3. Judson BL, Shaha AR. Nuclear Imaging and Minimally Invasive Surgery in the Management of Hyperparathyroidism. Journal of Nuclear Medicine: Official Publication, Society of Nuclear Medicine. 2008;49(11):10.2967/jnumed.107.050237.

4. Khan AA, Hanley DA, Rizzoli R, et al. Primary hyperparathyroidism: review and recommendations on evaluation, diagnosis, and management. A Canadian and international consensus. Osteoporosis International. 2017;28(1):1-19.
5. Lou I, Schneider DF, Sippel RS, Chen H, Elfenbein DM. The changing pattern of diagnosing primary hyperparathyroidism in young patients. American Journal of Surgery. 2017;213(1):146-50.
6. Pearce SH, Trump D, Wooding C, et al. Calcium-sensing receptor mutations in familial benign hypercalcemia and neonatal hyperparathyroidism. Journal of Clinical Investigation. 1995;96(6):2683-92.
7. Stokes VJ, Nielsen MF, Hannan FM, Thakker RV. Hypercalcemic disorders in children. Journal of Bone and Mineral Research. 2017;32(11):2157-70.

CHAPTER

17

Hyponatremia: Recent Approach to Management

Madhukar Mittal, Shobhith Shakya, Dinesh Kumar Singh

CASE

A 64-year-old male presents to the emergency with progressive altered behavior for 10 days, and seizures 1 day back. He is a known diabetic for 20 years and hypertensive. BP 140/90, RBS 130 mg, creatinine 1.2 mEq/L, Na 110 mEq/L, K 5.0.

There is no history of seizures and CT head is normal.

How would you evaluate this patient?

Q. 1 What other clinical history, examination and investigation would be relevant?

Ans.

History of:

- Vomiting, diarrhea,
- Drug intake (e.g. diuretics, etc.)
- Oliguria, swelling over feet or face
- Dyspnea, cardiac illness

Examination:

- Signs of dehydration (skin turgor, tongue, etc.)
- Anasarca
- Blood pressure (supine and postural)
- Pulse rate
- Systemic examination for cardiac, renal or liver disease
- Neurological examination

Investigation:

- Urinary sodium and creatinine
- Blood glucose
- Renal function
- Thyroid function
- Cortisol
- Plasma and urine osmolality.

Q. 2 What are the causes for hyponatremia?

Ans. *See* Flowchart 17.1

Hypovolemic	*Euvolemic*	*Hypervolemic*
Renal causes: • Diuretic excess • Mineralocorticoid deficiency • Salt-losing nephropathy • Cerebral salt wasting *Extrarenal loses:* • Vomiting • Diarrhea • Burns	• Glucocorticoid deficiency • Hypothyroidism • Stress/pain • Drugs • SIADH	• Renal failure • Nephrotic syndrome • Liver cirrhosis • Cardiac failure

Q. 3 What are the clinical manifestations of hyponatremia?

Ans.

Mild	*Moderate*	*Severe*
Anorexia, headache, nausea, vomiting, lethargy	Personality changes, muscle cramps, weakness, confusion, ataxia	Drowsiness, diminished reflexes, convulsions, coma

Q. 4 How would you approach a case of hyponatremia?

Ans. *See* Flowchart 17.2

Q. 5 What are the types of hyponatremia?

Ans. *See* Table 17.1, Flowcharts 17.1 and 17.3

FLOWCHART 17.1 Differentiating the causes of hyponatremia

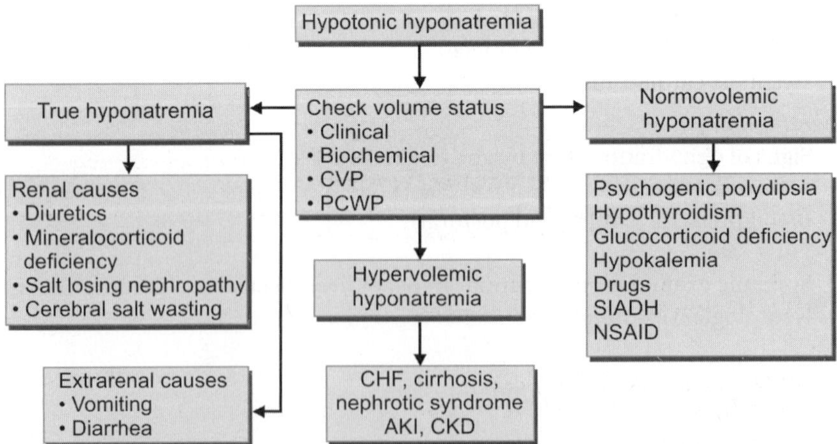

Abbreviations: CHF, congestive heart failure; AKI, acute kidney injury; CKD, chronic kidney disease; SIADH, syndrome of inappropriate antidiuretic hormone secretion; NSAID, nonsteroidal anti-inflammatory drug; CVP, central venous pressure; PCWP, pulmonary capillary wedge pressure

FLOWCHART 17.2 Approach to a case of hyponatremia

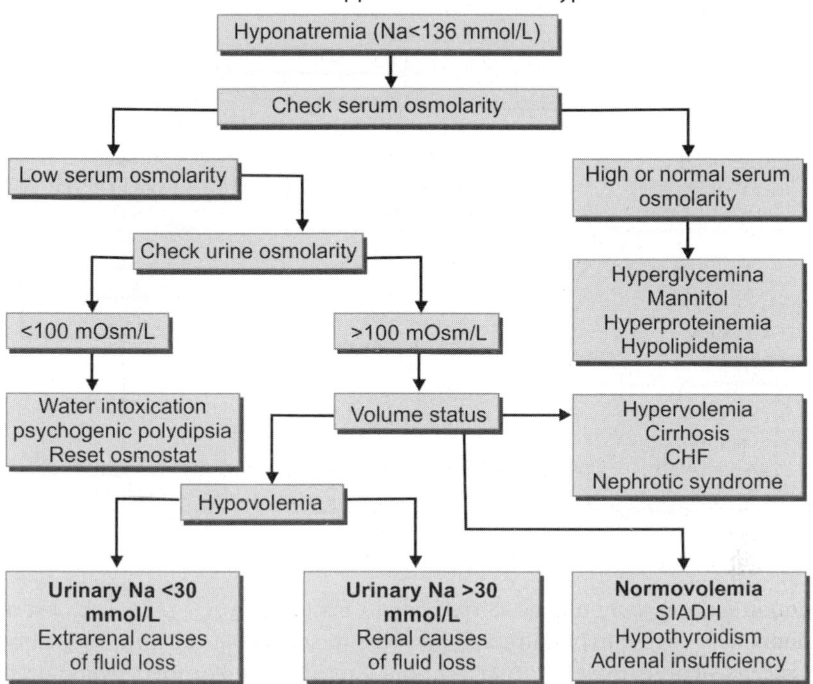

TABLE 17.1 Classification of hyponatremia by plasma tonicity

	Serum sodium concentration (mmol/L)	*Plasma osmolality (mOsm/kg H_2O)*	*Typical causes*
Hypotonic	<135	Low (<280)	SIADH; heart failure; cirrhosis
Isotonic	<135	Normal (280–295)	Hyperglycemia; pseudohyponatremia (hyperlipidemia, hyperproteinemia)
Hypertonic	<135	High (>295)	Severe hyperglycemia with dehydration; mannitol

Abbreviations: H_2O, water; kg, kilogram; L, liter; mmol, millimole; mOsm, milliosmole; SIADH, syndrome of inappropriate antidiuretic hormone secretion

Q. 6 What is the treatment of hyponatremia?

Ans.

- When hypovolemic, 0.9% saline
- When hypervolemic, fluid restriction and sometimes a loop diuretic
- When euvolemic, treatment of the cause
- When severe hyponatremia, cautious correction with hypertonic (3%) saline.

Rapid correction of hyponatremia, even mild hyponatremia, risks neurologic complications. Except possibly during the first few hours of treatment of severe

FLOWCHART 17.3 Pseudohyponatremia

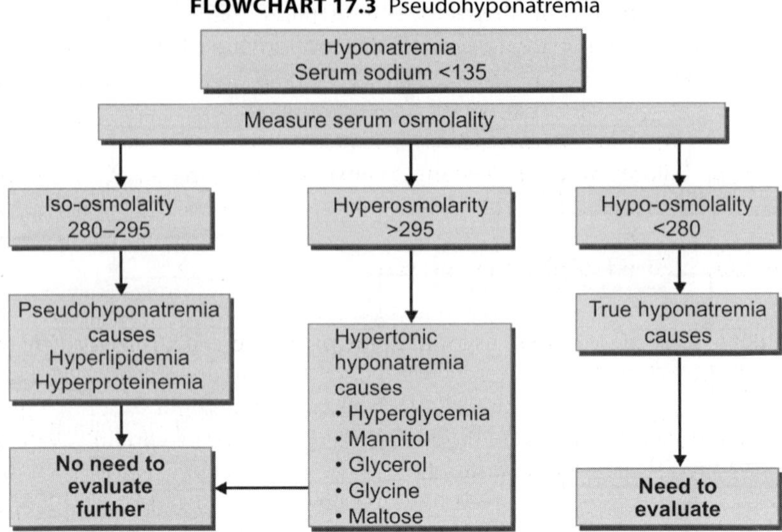

hyponatremia, Na should be corrected no faster than 0.5 mEq/L/h. Even in patients with severe hyponatremia, increase in serum Na concentration should not exceed 10 mEq/L over the first 24 hours. Any identified cause of hyponatremia is treated concurrently.

Mild hyponatremia: Mild, asymptomatic hyponatremia (i.e. serum Na>130 mEq/L) requires no saline because small adjustments are generally sufficient. In diuretic-induced hyponatremia, elimination of the diuretic may be enough; some patients need some Na replacement orally. Similarly, when mild hyponatremia results from inappropriate hypotonic parenteral fluid administration in patients with impaired water excretion, merely altering fluid therapy may suffice.

In patients with *hypovolemia* and normal adrenal function, administration of 0.9% saline usually corrects both hyponatremia and hypovolemia.

In *hypervolemic patients*, in whom hyponatremia is due to renal Na retention (e.g. heart failure, cirrhosis, nephrotic syndrome) and dilution, water restriction combined with treatment of the underlying disorder is required. In patients with heart failure, an ACE inhibitor, in conjunction with a loop diuretic, can correct refractory hyponatremia. In other patients in whom simple fluid restriction is ineffective, a loop diuretic in escalating doses can be used, sometimes in conjunction with IV 0.9% normal saline. Potassium and other electrolytes lost in the urine must be replaced. When hyponatremia is more severe and unresponsive to diuretics, intermittent or continuous hemofiltration may be needed to control ECF volume while hyponatremia is corrected with IV 0.9% normal saline.

In *euvolemia,* treatment is directed at the cause (e.g. hypothyroidism, adrenal insufficiency). When SIADH is present, water restriction (e.g. 250 to 500 mL/24 h) is generally required. Additionally, a loop diuretic may be combined with IV 0.9% saline as in hypervolemic hyponatremia. Lasting correction depends on successful treatment of the underlying disorder. When the underlying disorder is not correctable and severe water restriction is not possible, demeclocycline (300–600 mg po q12 hour) may be helpful by inducing a concentrating defect in the kidneys. However, demeclocycline may cause acute renal failure which is usually reversible when the drug is stopped. Intravenous conivaptan, an ADH receptor antagonist, causes effective water diuresis without significant loss of electrolytes in the urine and can be used in hospitalized patients for treatment of resistant hyponatremia.

Severe hyponatremia: Severe hyponatremia (serum Na < 120 mEq/L; effective osmolality < 238 mOsm/kg) in asymptomatic patients can be treated safely with stringent restriction of water intake. When neurologic symptoms (e.g. confusion, lethargy, seizures, coma) are present, IV 3% hypertonic saline should be given. The pace and degree of hyponatremia correction should be carefully watched. Serum Na should be raised no faster than 1 mEq/L/h, but replacement rates of up to 2 mEq/L/hour for the first 2–3 hours may be given for patients with seizures. However, the rise should be ≤10–12 mEq/L over the first 24 hour. More rapid correction risks precipitation of osmotic demyelination syndrome.

Hypertonic (3%) saline (containing 513 mEq Na/L) may be used, with frequent (q 2–4 h) electrolyte determinations. For patients with seizures or coma, ≤100 mL/h may be administered over 4–6 hours in amounts sufficient to raise the serum Na by 4–6 mEq/L.

Sodium correction: This amount (in mEq) may be calculated using the Na deficit formula as (Desired change in Na^+) × TBW (where TBW is 0.6 × body weight in kg in men and 0.5 × body weight in kg in women).

For example, the amount of Na needed to raise the Na from 104 to 110 in a 70 kg man can be calculated as follows:

(110 mEq/L – 104 mEq/L) × (0.6 L/kg × 70 kg) = 252 mEq

There is 513 mEq/L of Na in hypertonic saline, roughly 0.5 L of hypertonic saline is needed to raise the Na from 104 mEq/L to 110 mEq/L. This should be given over the succeeding 24 hours.

Adjustments may be needed based on serum Na^+ concentrations, which are monitored closely during the first few hours of treatment. Patients with seizures, coma, or altered mental status need supportive treatment, which may involve endotracheal intubation, mechanical ventilation, and treatment for seizures.

Q. 7 What are the recent advances in the management of hyponatremia?

Ans. The selective vasopressin (V_2) receptor antagonists conivaptan (IV) and tolvaptan (oral) are relatively new treatment options for severe or resistant hyponatremia. These drugs are to be used with caution because they may correct serum Na concentration too rapidly; they are typically reserved for severe (<120 mEq/L) and/or symptomatic hyponatremia that is resistant to correction with fluid restriction and for short-term use. The same rate of correction as for fluid restriction, ≤10 mEq/L over 24 hour, is used. These drugs should not be used for hypovolemic hyponatremia or in advanced chronic kidney disease.

Q. 8 What is syndrome of inappropriate antidiuretic hormone secretion (SIADH)?

Ans. It is a syndrome of renal sodium loss and hyponatremia resulting from inappropriate secretion of antidiuretic hormone.

Diagnostic criteria for SIADH:

Essential criteria:

- Effective serum osmolality <275 mOsm/kg
- Urine osmolality >100 mOsm/kg at some level of decreased effective osmolality
- Urine sodium concentration >30 mmol/L with normal dietary salt and water intake
- Clinical euvolemia
- Absence of adrenal, thyroid, pituitary or renal insufficiency
- No recent use of diuretic agents

Supplemental criteria:

- Serum uric acid <4 mg/dL
- Serum urea <21.6 mg/dL
- Failure to correct hyponatremia after 0.9% saline infusion
- Fractional sodium excretion >0.5%
- Fractional urea excretion >55%
- Fractional uric acid excretion >12%
- Correction of hyponatremia through fluid restriction

Q. 9 What are the causes of SIADH ?

Ans.

Malignant diseases	*Pulmonary disorders*	*Disorders of nervous system*
Carcinoma 1. Lung 2. Stomach 3. Pancreas 4. Bladder Lymphomas Sarcomas	Infections 1. Bacterial pneumonia 2. Viral pneumonia 3. Lung abscess 4. Tuberculosis 5. Aspergillosis Cystic fibrosis	Infections 1. Encephalitis 2. Meningitis 3. Brain abscess Subarachnoid hemorrhage Brain tumors Head trauma Hydrocephalus

Drugs	*Other causes*
Anticonvulsants 1. Carbamazepine 2. Sodium valproate Antidepressants 1. SSRIs 2. Tricyclics Antipsychotics 1. Phenothiazines Anticancer drugs 1. Cyclophosphamide 2. Vinca alkaloids	Hereditary 1. Gain-of-function mutation of vasopressin V2 receptor Idiopathic Transient 1. General anesthesia 2. Nausea 3. Pain 4. Stress

Q. 10 What is cerebral salt wasting syndrome (CSW)?

Ans. It is a syndrome in which patients with cerebral disease present with hyponatremia along with the presence of polyuria, elevated urinary sodium levels, and dehydration despite the presence of a low serum sodium concentration and adequate fluid intake (Table 17.2 and Fig. 17.1).

TABLE 17.2 Differences between SIADH and CSW

	CSW	*SIADH*
Plasma volume	↓	↑
Salt balance	Negative	Variable
Syndrome of dehydration	Present	Absent
Urine volume	Normal or ↑	Normal or ↓
Weight	↓	↑ or no change
CVP	↓	↑ or normal
PCWP	↓	↑ or normal
HCT	↑	↓ or no change
BUN:creatinine ratio	↑	Normal
S protein concentration	↑	Normal
Urine Na concentration	↑ ↑	↑
Serum K concentration	↑ or no change	↓ or no change
Serum uric acid concentration	Normal	↓
Treatment	Salt and fluid replacement	Fluid restriction

Abbreviations: SIADH, syndrome of inappropriate antidiuretic hormone secretion, HCT, hematocrit; CSW, cerebral salt-wasting; BUN, blood urea nitrogen

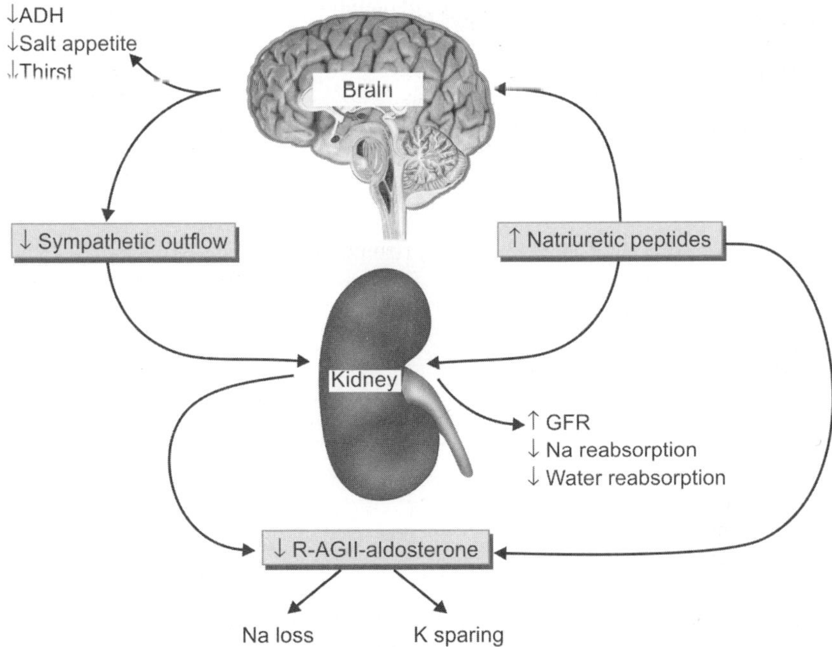

FIG. 17.1 Pathophysiology of cerebral salt wasting

Causes:
- Aneurysmal SAH
- Head trauma
- Central nervous system (CNS) malignancy
- Central nervous system (CNS) infections
- Postoperative neurosurgical setting.

SUGGESTED READING

1. Ball SG, Iqbal Z. Diagnosis and treatment of hyponatraemia. Best Pract Res Clin Endocrinol Metab. 2016;30(2):161-73. doi: 10.1016/j.beem.2015.12.001. Review. PubMed PMID: 27156756.
2. Drake-Holland AJ, Noble MI. The Hyponatremia Epidemic: A Frontier Too Far?Front Cardiovasc Med. 2016;3:35. Review. PubMed PMID: 27774451; PubMedCentral PMCID: PMC5053982.
3. Guillaumin J, DiBartola S. Disorders of sodium and water homeostasis. Vet Clin North Am Small Anim Pract. 2016 Dec 22. pii: S0195-5616(16)30133-4. doi:10.1016/j.cvsm.2016.10.015. [Epub ahead of print] Review. PubMed PMID: 28017410.
4. Hoorn EJ. Intravenous fluids: balancing solutions. J Nephrol. 2016 Nov 29.[Epub ahead of print] Review. PubMed PMID: 27900717.
5. Mocan M, Terheş LM, Blaga SN. Difficulties in the diagnosis and management of hyponatremia. Clujul Med. 2016;89(4):464-469. Review. PubMed PMID: 27857513; PubMed Central PMCID: PMC5111484.
6. Weismann D, Schneider A, Höybye C. Clinical aspects of symptomatichyponatremia. Endocr Connect. 2016;5(5):R35-R43. Review. PubMed PMID:27609587.
7. Zhang R, Wang S, Zhang M, Cui L. Hyponatremia in patients with chronic kidney disease. Hemodial Int. 2016 Jun 27. doi: 10.1111/hdi.12447. [Epub ahead of print] Review. PubMed PMID: 27350025.

CHAPTER

18

Pregnancy and Diabetes Mellitus

Rajeshwari Janakiraman

CASE

A 32-year-old lady office secretary of Indian origin with history of polycystic ovarian syndrome has conceived by ovulation induction. Her dad has hypertension and her mother has diabetes for 12 years. On examination, she is 160 cm, weighs 76 kg, and physical examination shows acanthosis, hirsutism, her BP is 120/70 mm Hg. Other systemic examination is unremarkable. She is seen by another obstetrician at 10 weeks of gestation and is advised oral glucose tolerance.

Q. 1 What is the definition of diabetes in pregnancy?

Ans. Varying degree of glucose intolerance diagnosed or recognized for the first time during pregnancy is gestational diabetes. It may be associated with other components of metabolic syndrome independent of other factors in the next 3 years. However, in recent days type 2 diabetes is seen in adolescent and young adults making it possible that type 2 diabetes is recognized first time during screening in pregnancy. Gestational diabetes mellitus accounts for 90% of cases of diabetes mellitus in pregnancy, while preexisting type 2 diabetes accounts for 8% of those diagnosed in pregnancy. In future this number is likely to increase.

Abnormal maternal glucose regulation occurs in 3–10% of pregnancies, the rising prevalence of diabetes mellitus—21 million people (7% of the population) have some form of diagnosed diabetes, another 6 million people may have undiagnosed diabetes and hence there is an expected increase in pregnancies with diabetes.

Q. 2 Why do sugars go high during pregnancy?

Ans. Normally in pregnancy the placental steroid and peptide hormones (e.g. estrogens, progesterone, and chronic somatomammotropin) raise linearly throughout the second and third trimesters. In pregnancy, human placental lactogen, which is structurally similar to growth hormone, and tumor-necrosis factor-alpha induce changes in the insulin receptor and in post-receptor signaling. Changes in the beta-subunit of the insulin receptor, decreased phosphorylation of tyrosine kinase on the insulin receptor, and alterations in insulin receptor substrate-1 (IRS-1) and the intracytoplasmic phosphatidylinositol 3-kinase (PI3K) appear to be involved in reducing glucose uptake in skeletal muscle tissue.

As a consequence, there is an increase in tissue insulin resistance; there is an increase in insulin secretion with feeding which escalates progressively during pregnancy. By the third trimester, 24-hour mean insulin levels are 50% higher than in the nonpregnant state.

In normoglycemic pregnant women, there is a tendency for hypoglycemia (plasma glucose mean = 65–75 mg/dL) in fasting and postabsorptive phases. This is because the fetus continues to transfer glucose across the placenta from the maternal bloodstream, even during periods of fasting irrespective of maternal glucose. Hypoglycemia becomes increasingly severe in postabsorptive state as pregnancy progresses as the glucose demand of the fetus increases.

In contrast to this, in glucose intolerant pregnant women as in polycystic ovary syndrome (PCOS) or metabolic syndrome, the beta cells may fail to meet this demand leading to impaired glucose tolerance.

This typically manifests as recurrent postprandial hyperglycemic episodes. These postprandial episodes are the most significant source of the accelerated growth exhibited by the fetus.

Q. 3 What are the normal blood glucose levels in pregnant women?

Ans. Using continuous glucose monitoring system (CGMS) in pregnant women the mean FBS was noted to be 75 +/– 12 mg/dL and the mean blood glucose level was 83.7 +/– 18 mg/dL with a postprandial peak glucose level of 110 +/– 16 mg/dL. The time interval to reach peak postprandial glucose level was 70 +/– 13 minutes with no significant difference between obese and normal weight pregnant women, and the peak glucose was higher and a delayed peak was seen in obese.

Q. 4 Why should we monitor blood glucose levels?

Ans. The prevalence of gestational diabetes is strongly related to the patient's race and culture. Prevalence rates are higher in black, Hispanic, Native American, and Asian women than in white women. For example, typically, only 1.5–2% of white women develop gestational diabetes mellitus, whereas Native Americans from the southwestern United States may have rates as high as 15%. In Hispanic, black and Asian populations, the incidence are 5–8%. Hence, high-risk population should be screened for gestational diabetes.

Q. 5 What are the risks to the pregnancy due to diabetes?

Ans. Maternal complications consist of hypertension, pre-eclampsia, increased risk of cesarean delivery, and development of diabetes mellitus after pregnancy. Fetal complications include macrosomia, neonatal hypoglycemia, polycythemia, increased perinatal mortality, congenital malformation, hyperbilirubinemia, respiratory distress syndrome, and hypocalcemia. Long-term consequences of macrosomia include increased risk of glucose intolerance, diabetes, and obesity in childhood.

The Australian Carbohydrate Intolerance Study in Pregnant Women (ACHOIS) was a large randomized control trial that investigated the role of screening and treatment of gestational diabetes in reducing perinatal complications, improving maternal outcomes, and affecting quality of life. This trial of 1000 participants showed a composite reduction in serious perinatal morbidity and mortality (death, shoulder dystocia, bone fracture, and nerve palsy) in the intervention group compared to the conventional group. Also, a decrease in prevalence in macrosomia in the intervention group infants and reduced rate of gestational hypertension in the intervention group was found.

Another large, multicenter randomized controlled trial conducted in the United States recruited women with mild gestational diabetes mellitus. One group received treatment consisting of dietary changes, self-monitoring of blood glucose and insulin if needed and the other received the usual prenatal care. Outcomes with respect to perinatal and obstetrical outcomes were compared. This trial of 19,665 participants used slightly different parameters to diagnose gestational diabetes mellitus but had similar outcomes. There was a significant reduction in macrosomia with the treatment group as well as reduction in rates of cesarean delivery, shoulder dystocia, pre-eclampsia or gestational hypertension and weight gain.

Finally, the HAPO (Hyperglycemia and Adverse Pregnancy Outcomes) trial, which included over 23,000 pregnant women, sought to clarify risks of adverse outcomes associated with various degrees of maternal glucose intolerance less severe than overt diabetes mellitus. The study results showed positive linear correlations between increasing levels of fasting, 1-hour and 2-hour plasma glucose after oral glucose tolerance testing (OGTT), and macrosomia and cord-blood C-peptide levels above the 90th percentile. Weaker associations were noted between glucose levels and cesarean delivery and neonatal hypoglycemia. The secondary outcomes of premature delivery, shoulder dystocia, hyperbilirubinemia, and pre-eclampsia were also noted to increase in incidence with higher levels of post OGTT glucose levels.

The HAPO trial showed that maternal, fetal, and neonatal outcomes increased significantly with maternal hyperglycemia even at lower threshold ranges than prior diagnostic criteria for GDM. This prompted the International Association of Diabetes and Pregnancy Study Groups (IADPSG), whose committee consists of members from US and International diabetes organizations, including American Diabetes Association (ADA), and obstetrical organizations, to revise recommendations for diagnosing GDM. Whereas previously in the 2005 Fifth International Workshop-Conference on Gestational Diabetes Mellitus screening was based on risk stratification, now the IADPSG along with the ADA recommend that all women with no prior history of diabetes undergo 75-g glucose oral glucose tolerance test (OGTT) at 24–28 weeks gestation.

Race also influences many complications of diabetes mellitus in pregnancy. For instance, black women have been shown to have lower rates of macrosomia, despite similar levels of glycemic control. Conversely, Hispanic women have higher rates of macrosomia and birth injury than women of other ethnicity, even with aggressive management.

Infants of mothers with preexisting diabetes (T1 or T2) experience double the risk of serious injury at birth, triple the likelihood of cesarean delivery, and quadruple the incidence of newborn intensive care unit (NICU) admission. Studies indicate that the risk of these morbidities is directly proportional to the degree of maternal hyperglycemia.

FETAL RISKS

Miscarriages

Pre-existing diabetes mellitus, miscarriage rate is about 9–14%. There is a strong association between the glycemic control at early pregnancy and the miscarriage rate. Poor glycemic control has been shown to doubles the early fetal loss in women with diabetes. A correlation also exists between chronic diabetes complications and miscarriage rates.

Patients with long-standing (>10 years) and poorly controlled diabetes (glycosylated hemoglobin exceeding 11%) have been shown to have a miscarriage rate of up to 44%, with nephropathy, and other microvascular complications. With excellent glycemic control, the miscarriage rates can be reduced to background population rates.

Malformations

As compared to population risk of major birth defects of 1–2%, women with overt and poorly controlled diabetes glycemic control before conception, the likelihood of a anomalies is increased 4- to 8-times. Though it was estimated to be as high as 18% in women with preexisting diabetes mellitus, more recent studies, in patients who received better preconception care and first trimester management, report anomaly rates between 5.1% and 9.8%.

Anomalies: Cardiovascular and neurological anomalies form two-thirds of the defects seen. Neural tubal defects are about 20 times more than general population. Other anomalies affect genitourinary, skeletal and gastrointestinal abnormalities. Sacral agenesis is considered pathognomonic of preexisting diabetes.

It is interesting that paternal diabetes does not increase fetal anomalies proving that maternal or intrauterine environment is the sole cause for this.

When the first-trimester maternal glycosylated hemoglobin values was of less than 8.5%, the anomaly rate was only 3.4% in contrast to that it was 22.4% with poorer glycemic control in the periconceptional period (HbA_{1c} >8.5%). An overall malformation rate of 13.3% was reported in 105 patients with diabetes, but the risk of delivering a malformed infant was comparable to a normal population when the HbA_{1c} was less than 7%. More recently, in a review of 7 cohort studies, researchers found that patients with a normal glycosylated hemoglobin, the absolute risk of an anomaly were 2%. At 2 SD above normal, this risk was 3%, with an odds ratio of 1.2 (1.1–1.4). There was a direct relationship of anomalies with HbA_{1c}.

Trials comparing a pre-conceptional intensive metabolic program to standard treatment have demonstrated lowered rates of perinatal mortality (0% vs 7%) and congenital anomalies (2% vs 14%). In addition, when the preconceptional counseling program was discontinued, the congenital anomaly rate increased by over 50%.

Macrosomia

Birth weight is determined by maternal factors like hyperglycemia, gestational age at delivery, maternal pre-pregnancy body mass index (BMI), maternal height, pregnancy weight gain, the presence of hypertension, and cigarette smoking.

Macrosomia defined as a birth weight above the 90th percentile for gestational age or greater than 4000 g. Macrosomia occurs in 15–45% of babies born to diabetic women, a 3-fold increase from normoglycemic controls. Apart from that maternal obesity is a strong and independent factor for fetal macrosomia.

When women who are very obese (weight > 300 lb) were compared with women of normal weight, the newborns of obese women had more than double the risk of macrosomia compared to those of women of normal weight. This may explain the failure of glycemic control to completely prevent fetal macrosomia in several series.

Excess nutrient delivery to the fetus causes macrosomia and truncal fat deposition, but whether fasting or peak glucose values are more correlated with fetal overgrowth is less clear. Data from the diabetes in Early Pregnancy Project indicate that fetal birth weight correlates best with second- and third-trimester postprandial blood sugar levels and not with fasting or mean glucose levels. When postprandial glucose values average 120 mg/dL or less, approximately 20% of infants can be expected to be macrosomic. When postprandial levels range as high as 160 mg/dL, macrosomia rates can reach 35%.

Macrosomia is associated with excessive rates of neonatal morbidity. The infants of diabetic mothers have been shown to have 5-fold higher rates of severe hypoglycemia, a 4-fold increase in macrosomia, and a doubled increase in neonatal jaundice relative to infants of mothers without diabetes.

The macrosomic fetus in diabetic pregnancy develops a unique pattern of overgrowth with central deposition of subcutaneous fat in the abdominal and interscapular areas.

Neonates of diabetic mothers have a larger shoulder and extremity circumference, a decreased head-to-shoulder ratio, significantly higher body fat, and thicker upper limb skin folds compared with nondiabetic control infants of similar weights. Because fetal head size is not increased during poorly controlled diabetic pregnancy, but shoulder and abdominal girth are markedly enhanced. This leads to the risk of injury peripartum injury (e.g. Erb palsy).

Thus, birth injury, including shoulder dystocia and brachial plexus trauma, are more common among infants of diabetic mothers, and macrosomic fetuses are at the highest risk.

The Australian Carbohydrate Intolerance Study in Pregnant Women (ACHOIS) trial showed a positive correlationship between severity of maternal fasting hyperglycemia and risk of shoulder dystocia, with a 1 mmol increase in fasting glucose leading to a 2.09 relative risk for shoulder dystocia.

In addition, there appears to be a role for excessive fetal insulin levels in mediating accelerated fetal growth. In a study done to compare umbilical cord sera in infants of diabetic mothers and controls, the heavier, fatter babies from diabetic pregnancies were also hyperinsulinemic.

Serial fetal ultrasonography of women with diabetes shows that the growth velocity of the abdominal circumference is often well above the growth percentiles as compared to fetuses with nondiabetic mother. Abdominal circumference is indeed higher than the fetal head and femur percentiles. The growth of the abdominal circumference begins to rise significantly above normal after 24 weeks. If oral glucose tolerance is normal, but follow-up scan show an abnormal percentiles of abdominal circumference, more closer monitoring blood glucose levels is worthwhile.

Intrauterine Growth Retardation

Though most fetuses of mothers with uncontrolled diabetes have macrosomia, growth retardation occurs in fetuses of women with pre-existing diabetes. The most important predictor of fetal growth restriction is underlying chronic vascular disease. Fetuses of women with diabetes-associated microvascular complications especially nephropathy and retinopathy and/or chronic hypertension are most at risk for growth restriction.

Perinatal Complications

With improvement in healthcare and availability of diabetes medications especially insulin pre-pregnancy counseling and preconception management, the diabetic pregnancy outcomes have improved over years.

Birth Trauma

Injuries during delivery including shoulder dystocia and brachial plexus injury are more common among macrosomic infants of diabetic mothers especially with difficult vaginal delivery and shoulder dystocia. The incidence is 2 to 4 fold higher in women with diabetes as compared to nondiabetes pregnancies of 0.3–0.5%. Other common birth injuries include brachial plexus injury, facial nerve injury, and cephalhematoma. With strict glycemic control, these can be reduced (3.2 vs 2.5%).

Hypoglycemia

About 15–25% of neonates with diabetic mothers develop hypoglycemia during the immediate newborn period. Neonatal hypoglycemia is less frequent when tight glycemic control is maintained during pregnancy and even during labor. Dextrose infusions during labor increase the risk of neonatal hypoglycemia. Unrecognized postnatal hypoglycemia may lead to neonatal seizures, coma, brain damage and death.

Hypocalcemia

Up to 50% of infants of diabetic mothers have low levels of serum calcium (<7 mg/100 mL). These changes in calcium appear to be attributable to immaturity of parathyroid glands. With improved management of diabetes in pregnancy, the rate of neonatal hypocalcemia has been reduced to 5% or less.

Polycythemia

Hyperglycemia is a powerful stimulus to fetal erythropoietin production, mediated by decreased fetal oxygen tension. Untreated neonatal polycythemia may promote vascular sludging, ischemia, and infarction of vital organs like the kidneys and central nervous system.

Hyperbilirubinemia

Hyperbilirubinemia occurs in 2 times higher in neonates born of diabetic mothers; the causes include prematurity and polycythemia. Increased destruction of red blood cells contributes to the risk of jaundice and kernicterus.

Respiratory Distress Syndrome

In healthy pregnancy, fetus achieves pulmonary maturity at a mean gestational age of 34–35 weeks. By 37 weeks' gestation, more than 99% of healthy newborn infants have mature lung profiles as assessed by phospholipid assays. However, in a diabetic pregnancy, the risk of respiratory distress may not pass until after 38.5 gestational weeks. Added to this there is higher percentage of premature deliveries due to macrosomia and polyhydramnios.

With improved prenatal maternal glycemic control and newer concepts in timing and mode of delivery has resulted in a decline in RDS from 31% to 3%. Nevertheless, respiratory distress syndrome continues to be a relatively preventable complication. Steroid prophylaxis at appropriate timing prevents this to a great extent.

MATERNAL

Diabetes Complications

In type 1 diabetes mellitus the duration of diabetes may be long enough to have microvascular complications. Almost 50% of those with retinopathy prior to pregnancy will have worsening during pregnancy. In most of them, there is some degree of improvement postpartum. However, long-term progression is slower in these women due to better glycemic control.

During pregnancy GFR increases by 30–50% and microalbuminuria is common. In preexisting diabetes with nephropathy with deterioration in renal function, but rapid progression to ESRD is not seen. Preterm delivery, intrauterine growth retardation, and pre-eclampsia are all significantly more common in those with nephropathy.

Postrenal transplantation pregnancy is possible but will need a coordinated effort by multispecialty experts.

Hypertension

Chronic hypertension is common in patients with diabetes especially type 2. During pregnancy they are at high risk of worsening of control, intrauterine growth retardation, pre-eclampsia, abruption placenta and cardiovascular events. Women with advanced age, preexisting diabetes, or with renal or retinal involvement are at higher risk of chronic hypertension and pre-eclampsia.

Pre-eclampsia is more frequent among women with diabetes (approximately 12%) versus the nondiabetic population (8%). In one study, when the fasting plasma glucose (FPG) was <105 mg/dL, the rate of pre-eclampsia was 7.8%; with an FPG >105 mg/dL, the rate of pre-eclampsia was 13.8%.

The fetal and neonatal morbidity attributable to diabetes in pregnancy should be considered preventable with early diagnosis and effective treatment therapies.

Q. 6 If diabetes in pregnancy can cause so much havoc, can we prevent it?

Ans. The answer is yes and the first step is to suspect and diagnose diabetes during pregnancy. Screening for diabetes is a controversial issue. In 1995, Mosses proposed universal screening for gestational diabetes. With universal screening gestational diabetes mellitus was diagnosed in 6.7% of the women overall, in 8.5% of the women aged 30 years or older, in 12.3% of the women with a preconception body mass index of 30 kg/m^2 or greater, and in 11.6% of women with a family history of diabetes in a first-degree relative and presence of hypertension before pregnancy or during early pregnancy. Gestational diabetes mellitus was present in 4.8% of the women without risk factors. In races where the risk is the incidence of gestational diabetes is low it may not be cost-effective.

Hence, it may not be practicable in all populations. So a risk stratified approach has been suggested. The diagnostic methods itself was controversial until recently. From the above study, we can deduce that high preconceptional body mass index (>30 kg/m^2), older women (>30 years), and family history of diabetes are at risk.

The current recommendations from the American Diabetes Association "Standards of Medical Care in Diabetes—2017"—screen all women for risk factors during first antenatal visit. Very high higher grades of obesity, past history of gestational diabetes mellitus or delivery of an large for gestational age baby, presence of glycosuria and history of polycystic ovarian syndrome and strong family history of type 2 diabetes. For all others screening at 24–28 weeks is recommended and repeat screening for high-risk women whose glucose tolerance was normal in first screening test.

It may be avoided in women whose risk of gestational diabetes is very low (aged <25 years, belongs to a race with low risk for diabetes, no family history of diabetes and previous pregnancies were normoglycemia with good obstetric outcome).

The Endocrine Society recommends that all pregnant women at risk but who are not yet diagnosed with diabetes should be screened for the disease with a fasting plasma glucose (FPG), an HbA_{1c}, or a random plasma glucose test at their first prenatal visit. A fasting plasma glucose of 126 mg/dL or higher (≥7.0 mmol/L), a random plasma glucose of 200 mg/dL or higher (≥11.1 mmol/L), or an HbA_{1c} of 6.5% or higher indicates overt diabetes (type 1, type 2, or other), while an FPG of 92–125 mg/dL (5.1–6.9 mmol/L) indicates gestational diabetes.

A diagnosis of overt diabetes must be confirmed with a second test (FPG, untimed random plasma glucose, HbA_{1c}, or oral glucose tolerance test [OGTT]); these must be performed when hyperglycemic symptoms are absent and must be abnormal on another day. At 24–28 weeks' gestation, a result of 153–199 mg/dL (8.5–11 mmol/L) for a 2-hour, 75-g OGTT indicates gestational diabetes, while a test result of 200 mg/dL or higher (≥11.1 mmol/L) indicates overt diabetes.

Whatever is the type of diabetes, the principles of treatment would be the same, but postnatal follow-up and treatment may be modified.

Screening Tools for Gestational Diabetes

The best method for screening for gestational diabetes continues to be controversial. The 2-step system is currently recommended in the United States. A 50-g, 1-hour glucose challenge test (GCT) is followed by a 100-g, 3-hour OGTT for those with an abnormal screening result. Alternatively, for high-risk women, proceeding directly to the 100-g, 3-hour OGTT can use a one-step approach.

American Diabetes Association Recommendations

The sensitivity of gestational diabetes mellitus testing depends on the threshold value used for the 50-g glucose challenge. Current recommendations from the American Diabetes Association "Standards of Medical Care in Diabetes—2017" and the American College of Obstetricians and Gynecologists (ACOG) note that a threshold value of 140 mg/dL after 75 g oral glucose results in approximately 80% detection of gestational diabetes, whereas a threshold of 130 mg/dL results in 90% detection. A potential disadvantage of using the lower value of 130 mg/dL is an approximate doubling in the number of OGTTs performed.

In updated guidelines, the American Diabetes Association recommends use of either the 1-step or the 2-step screening method (recommended by the National Institutes of Health), advising that both tests are acceptable screens.

Oral Glucose Tolerance Test

The patient should remain seated during the test, and should not smoke.

Diagnosis of GDM is made if any of the following plasma glucose values are exceeded after 75 gram glucose is given:

- Fasting of 92 mg/dL or higher (5.1 mmol/L)
- One-hour of 180 mg/dL or higher (10 mmol/L)
- Two-hour of 153 mg/dL or higher (8.5 mmol/L)

Two-step Approach

Step 1: Perform a 50-g GLT (nonfasting), with plasma glucose measurement at 1 h, at 24–28 weeks of gestation in women not previously diagnosed with overt diabetes. If the plasma glucose level easured 1 h after the load is >130 mg/dL, proceed to a 100-g OGTT.

Step 2: The 100-g OGTT should be performed when the patient is fasting. The diagnosis of GDM is made if at least two of the following four plasma glucose levels (measured fasting and 1 h, 2 h, 3 h after the OGTT) are met or exceeded:

Carpenter/Coustan
Fasting 95 mg/dl
1 h 180 mg/dL
2 h 155 mg/dL
3 h 140 mg/dL

Q. 7 Will diabetes continue after pregnancy? If planned for another pregnancy will it recur?

Ans. The recurrence risk with future pregnancies has been reported to be as high as 68%. In addition, approximately one-third will develop overt diabetes mellitus within 5 years of delivery, with higher-risk ethnicity having risks nearing 50%.

Q. 8 How do we go about if the sugar levels are high?

Ans. Education is the cornerstone of effective metabolic management of the patient with diabetes during pregnancy. Especially, trained and certified nurses and dietitians (diabetes educators) are the most effective in achieving this.

- Initial treatment for gestational diabetes should consist of lifestyle changes with regard to diet and fitness.

If lifestyle changes cannot sufficiently control blood glucose, medications should be used.

If 2-hour postprandial glucose levels are maintained below 120 mg/dL, approximately 20% of fetuses demonstrate macrosomia. If postprandial levels range up to 160 mg/dL, macrosomia rates rise to 35%.

Pre-existing diabetes (type 1 or 2):

During the first trimester of pregnancy, women with diabetes should undergo testing (in addition to normal prenatal laboratory tests) for HbA_{1c}, blood urea nitrogen, serum creatinine, thyroid-stimulating hormone, and free thyroxine levels, as well as spot urine protein-to-creatinine ratio and capillary blood sugar levels 4–5 times daily as feasible.

Second-trimester testing for women with diabetes includes a repeat spot urine protein-to-creatinine study in women with elevated value in first trimester, a repeat HbA_{1c}, and capillary blood sugar levels 4–5 times daily.

In the first trimester, patients should have an ultrasonogram assessment (including measurement of crown-rump length) for pregnancy dating and viability. Consider nuchal translucency if the fetus is at high risk for cardiac defects (e.g. because of high maternal glycosylated hemoglobin).

In the second trimester, perform a detailed anatomy ultrasonogram at 18–20 weeks, and a fetal echocardiogram if the maternal glycosylated hemoglobin values were less than 8.5%.

In the third trimester, perform a growth ultrasonogram to assess fetal size every 4–6 weeks from 26 weeks to 36 weeks in women with overt preexisting diabetes. Perform a growth ultrasonogram for fetal size at least once at 36–37 weeks for women with gestational diabetes mellitus. Consider performing this study more frequently if macrosomia is suggested. If maternal diabetes is longstanding or associated with known microvascular disease, obtain a baseline maternal electrocardiogram (ECG) and echocardiogram.

If pre-eclampsia is suggested, order the following tests:

- 24-hour urine collection
- Blood urea nitrogen and serum creatinine
- Liver function tests
- Uric acid
- Complete blood cell count
- Assessment of fetal well-being with nonstress test, amniotic fluid index, fetal growth and Doppler ultrasonographic examination of the umbilical cord and middle cerebral artery.

An eye examination to look for diabetic retinopathy should be performed in women with type 1 or type 2 diabetes; if found, the retinopathy should be treated before conception.

In patients with preexisting diabetes, nutritional and metabolic intervention must be initiated and screen for microvascular complications well before pregnancy begins, because birth defects occur during the critical 3–6 weeks after conception.

Insulin remains the standard medication for treatment of diabetes during pregnancy, but the oral agents glibenclamide and metformin are increasingly used.

The long-term safety of oral agents in pregnancy is not known so insulin is the preferred option.

To reduce diabetes-associated neonatal morbidity, counsel the patient before conception and perform a medical risk assessment in all women with overt diabetes and those with a history of gestational diabetes mellitus during a previous pregnancy.

Key features of an effective diabetes management program include performing a thorough assessment of cardiovascular, renal, and ophthalmologic status; and instituting a regimen of frequent and regular monitoring of both preprandial and postprandial capillary glucose levels.

Controversy exists as to whether the target glucose levels to be maintained during diabetic pregnancy should be designed to limit macrosomia or to closely mimic nondiabetic pregnancy profiles. The Fifth International Workshop Conference on Gestational Diabetes recommends the following:

- Fasting plasma glucose less than 95 mg/dL
- One-hour postprandial plasma glucose less than 140 mg/dL, or
- Two-hour postprandial plasma glucose less than 120 mg/dL
- The goal of medical nutritional therapy is to avoid single large meals and those with a large proportion of simple carbohydrates. A total of 6 feedings per day is preferred, with 3 major meals and 3 snacks to limit the amount of energy intake at any time interval. The diet should include foods with complex carbohydrates and cellulose, such as whole grain breads and legumes
- Carbohydrates should account for less than 50% of the diet, with protein and fats equally accounting for the remainder. However, moderate restriction of carbohydrates to 35–40% has been shown to decrease maternal glucose levels and improve maternal and fetal outcomes
- Nutritional therapy should be supervised by a registered dietitian, with regular dietary assessment and counseling. For obese women (BMI >30 kg/m^2), a 30–33% calorie restriction (to 25 kcal/kg actual weight per day or less) has been shown to reduce hyperglycemia and plasma triglycerides with no increase in ketonuria.

The insulin regimen should result in a smooth glucose profile throughout the day, with no hypoglycemic reactions between meals or at night. Initiate the regimen early enough before pregnancy so that the glycosylated hemoglobin, level is lowered into the reference range for at least 3 months before conception. Any insulin regime-mixed split insulin or premixed insulin can be used to suit the patient.

Patients should take a prenatal vitamin containing at least 1 mg of folic acid daily for at least 3 months before conception to minimize the risk of neural tube defects in the fetus.

In an ideal world, diabetes-in-pregnancy programs would focus to reach to nonpregnant reproductive-aged women with diabetes in order to minimize the morbidity due to poor preconceptional control. Pre-emptively educate non-pregnant women to avoid pregnancy until their HbA_{1c} value is in within the reference range (<6.5%). Stop drugs like statins, ACE I, or ARBs that are contraindicated in pregnancy.

Team Care

Most large programs for treating women with diabetes during pregnancy have a staff that includes a registered nurse, a certified diabetes educator, a dietitian knowledgeable about pregnancy, and a social worker. Successful management of diabetic pregnancy is optimized when this type of team care is available.

Patients with preexisting diabetes require modification of their pharmacologic regimen to meet the changing metabolic demands of pregnancy. In gestational diabetes, early intervention with insulin or an oral agent is key to achieving a good outcome when diet therapy fails to provide adequate glycemic control. Determine the choice of insulin and regimen based on the patient's individual glucose profile.

The goal of insulin therapy during pregnancy is to achieve glucose profiles similar to those of nondiabetic pregnant women. Given that healthy pregnant women maintain their postprandial blood sugar excursions within a relatively narrow range (70–120 mg/dL), reproducing this profile requires meticulous daily attention by both the patient and clinician.

Insulins lispro, aspart, regular, and neutral protamine hagedorn (NPH) are well-studied in pregnancy and regarded as safe and effective. Insulin glargine is less well-studied, and given its long pharmacologic effect, may exacerbate periods of maternal hypoglycemia. Insulin detemir is safe and comparable to NPH insulin in pregnancy.

As pregnancy progresses, the increasing fetal demand for glucose and the progressive lowering of maternal fasting and between-meal blood sugar levels increases the risk of symptomatic hypoglycemia. Upward adjustment of short-acting insulin doses to control postprandial glucose surges within the target band only exacerbates the tendency to interprandial hypoglycemia. Thus, any insulin regimen for pregnant women requires combinations and timing of insulin injections quite different from those that are effective in the nonpregnant state. Further, the regimens must be continuously modified as the pregnancy progresses from the first to the third trimester and insulin resistance rises. However, when they have chronic hypertension or pregnancy-induced hypertension or placental insufficiency they may develop hypoglycemia.

In a select group of patients, use of an insulin pump may improve glycemic control while enhancing patient convenience. These devices can be programmed to infuse varying basal and bolus levels of insulin, which change smoothly even while the patient sleeps or is otherwise preoccupied.

The effectiveness of continuous subcutaneous insulin infusion in pregnancy is well-established. Similar HbA_{1c} levels, macrosomia rates, and cesarean rates in 33 pregnant women managed with insulin pump, compared with 23 receiving multiple insulin injections have been reported. No differences in glycemic control or perinatal outcome between 25 women treated with insulin pump in pregnancy and 68 women who received conventional insulin treatment were seen.

Oral Therapy

Glyburide

The efficacy and safety of insulin have made it the standard for treatment of diabetes during pregnancy. Nevertheless, the oral agents glyburide and metformin are gaining popularity. Trials have shown these agents to be effective and no evidence of harm to the fetus has been found, although the potential for long-term adverse effects remains a concern.

Glyburide is a second-generation sulfonylurea that is minimally transported across the human placenta. This is probably largely due to the high plasma protein binding coupled with a short half-life. In addition, a human placenta perfusion study demonstrated active glyburide transport from the fetus to the mother.

A 2000 randomized trial comparing glyburide to insulin in 404 pregnancies found no difference between the groups in mean maternal blood glucose levels, the percentage of infants who were LGA, birth weights, or neonatal complications. Only 4% of patients in the glyburide study arm required addition of insulin to achieve glucose control. Since this study, several prospective and retrospective studies involving more than 775 pregnancies have concluded glyburide is as safe and effective as insulin. All studies comparing glyburide to traditional insulin have demonstrated similar levels of glycemic control. Most studies show no differences in maternal or neonatal outcomes with glyburide.

Success rates for achieving glycemic control with glyburide vary from 79% to 86%. Studies evaluating predictors of failure with glyburide cite the following risk factors:

- Advanced maternal age
- Earlier gestational age at diagnosis
- Higher gravidity and parity
- Higher mean fasting glucose level.

Glyburide should not be used in the first trimester, because its effects, if any, on the embryo are unknown. In the past, teratogenic effects were seen with first-generation sulfonylurea, which readily crossed the placenta. Glyburide has been found to be associated with higher rates of neonatal hypoglycemia and macrosomia than insulin or metformin.

Metformin

Metformin is a biguanide, which functions mainly by decreasing hepatic glucose output. Metformin crosses the placenta, and umbilical cord levels have been shown to be even higher than maternal levels.

An initial retrospective study comparing glyburide, metformin, and insulin in pregnancy raised concern, because of increased rates of pre-eclampsia and perinatal mortality when metformin was used in the third trimester. It should be noted that in this study the patients on metformin had a higher body mass index and were older than the patients on glyburide or insulin. Since this initial study, however, several other prospective and retrospective studies involving over 300 pregnant patients have not confirmed the increased rates of pre-eclampsia or perinatal mortality. These subsequent studies have demonstrated similar efficacy, safety, and maternal and fetal outcomes with metformin.

As study compared the effect of metformin and glyburide in women with gestational diabetes who did not achieve glycemic control with diet. Between the 2 groups, patients who achieved glycemic control did not differ with regard to mean fasting and 2-hour postprandial blood glucose level. However, the percentage of women who did not achieve glycemic control and required insulin was 2.1 times higher with metformin (34.7%) than with glyburide (16.2%).

Metformin has been shown to cause a higher risk of prematurity as compared to insulin. Patients treated with oral agents should be informed that they cross the placenta and though no adverse effects on the fetus have been demonstrated long-term studies are lacking.

Prenatal Obstetric Management

Periodic Fetal Biophysical Testing

The goals of management of third-trimester pregnancies in women with diabetes are to prevent stillbirth and asphyxia while minimizing maternal and fetal morbidity associated with delivery. Monitoring fetal growth is essential to select the proper timing and route of delivery. This is accomplished by frequent testing for fetal well-being and serial ultrasonographic examinations to follow fetal size.

Various fetal biophysical tests are available to the clinician to ensure that the fetus is well oxygenated, including fetal heart rate testing, fetal movement assessment, ultrasonographic biophysical scoring, and fetal umbilical Doppler ultrasonographic studies. If applied properly, most of these tests can be used with confidence to provide assurance of fetal well-being while awaiting fetal maturity.

If the fetus is not macrosomic and the results of biophysical testing are reassuring, the obstetrician can await spontaneous labor. In patients with gestational diabetes mellitus and superb glycemic control, continued fetal testing and expectant management can be considered until 41 weeks' gestation. In the fetus with an abdominal circumference significantly larger than the head circumference or an estimated fetal weight above 4000 g, consider induction. After 40 or more weeks, the benefits of continued conservative management are likely to be outweighed by the danger of fetal compromise. Induction of labor before 41 weeks' gestation in pregnant women with diabetes, regardless of the readiness of the cervix, is prudent.

Comparing the outcomes associated with labor induction in patients with gestational diabetes at 38 weeks versus expectant management with fetal testing, Expectant management has been shown to increase gestational age at delivery by 1 week, but it did not significantly reduce the cesarean delivery. However, the prevalence of macrosomia was significantly greater among infants in the expectantly managed group (23%) than among those in the active induction group (10%). This suggests that routine induction of women with diabetes on or before 39 weeks' gestation does not increase the risk of cesarean delivery and may reduce the risk of macrosomia.

An optimal time for delivery of most diabetic pregnancies is typically on or after the 39th week. Deliver a patient with diabetes before 39 weeks' gestation only for maternal or fetal indications.

Because the risk of shoulder dystocia and fetal injury in labor is increased 3-fold in diabetic pregnancy, elective cesarean section should be considered if the fetus is suspected to be significantly obese.

Q. 9 How is intrapartum glycemic management planned for this lady?

Ans. Maintenance of intrapartum metabolic homeostasis optimizes postnatal infant transition by reducing neonatal hyperinsulinemia and subsequent hypoglycemia. Those women who were controlled with diet and lifestyle changes alone do not need close monitoring peripartum. In these women avoiding dextrose in intravenous fluids normally maintains excellent blood glucose control. After 1–2 hours of monitoring, no further assessments of capillary blood sugar typically are necessary.

But watch for hypoglycemia. The use of a combined insulin and glucose infusion during labor to maintain maternal blood sugars in a narrow range (80–110 mg/dL) is a common and clinically efficient practice. Typical infusion rates are 5% dextrose in Ringer lactate solution at 100 mL/h and regular insulin at 0.5–1.0 U/h. Capillary blood sugar levels are monitored hourly in these patients. Immediate postpartum blood glucose tends to drop and most women need only dextrose containing solution postdelivery until they are ready for ingesting meal.

Q. 10 What postpartum care will be needed for this lady?

Ans. The diabetes-in-pregnancy team is also able to help the patient during the puerperal period with the challenges of lactation, diet, sleep, and glycemic control. This team is also most effective in providing a smooth return to nonpregnant metabolic management. Initial follow-up at 6 weeks to 6 months with oral glucose tolerance test is recommended. Following that, these patients should have lifelong screening for prediabetes or diabetes development every 3 years.

SUGGESTED READING

1. American College of Obstetricians and Gynecologists. Screening and diagnosis of gestational diabetes mellitus. Committee Opinion No. 504. American College of Obstetricians and Gynecologists. Obstet Gynecol. 2011;118:751-3.

2. American Diabetes Association. Management of Diabetes in Pregnancy: Standards of Medical Care in Diabetes-2018. Diabetes Care. 2018;41(Suppl 1):S137-43.
3. Crowther CA, Hiller JE, Moss JR, McPhee AJ, Jeffries WS, Robinson JS. Effect of treatment of gestational diabetes mellitus on pregnancy outcomes. N Engl J Med. 2005;352(24):2477-86. [Medline].
4. Jovanovic L, Pettitt DJ. Gestational diabetes mellitus. JAMA. 2001;286(20):2516-8. [Medline].
5. Landon MB, Spong CY, Thom E, Carpenter MW, Ramin SM, Casey B. A multicenter, randomized trial of treatment for mild gestational diabetes. N Engl J Med. 2009;361(14):1339-48. [Medline].
6. Lowe LP, Metzger BE, Dyer AR, Lowe J, McCance DR, Lappin TR, et al. Hyperglycemia and Adverse Pregnancy Outcome (HAPO) Study: associations of maternal A1C and glucose with pregnancy outcomes. Diabetes Care. 2012;35(3):574-80. [Medline]. [Full Text].
7. Metzger BE, Buchanan TA. Summary and Recommendations of the Fifth International Workshop-Conference on Gestational Diabetes Mellitus. Diabetes Care. 2005;30 (Suppl 2):S251-260.
8. Metzger BE, Coustan DR. Proceedings of the Fourth International Work-shop-Conference on Gestational Diabetes Mellitus. Diabetes Care. 1998;21(Suppl 2): B1-B167.
9. Metzger BE, Gabbe SG, Persson B, Buchanan TA, Catalano PA. International association of diabetes and pregnancy study groups recommendations on the diagnosis and classification of hyperglycemia in pregnancy. Diabetes Care. 2010;33(3):676-82. [Medline].
10. National Diabetes Information. Clearinghouse (NDIC). *http://diabetes.niddk.nih.gov/DM/PUBS/statistics/#Gestational.* 2011.
11. Setji TL, Brown AJ, Feinglos MN. Gestational Diabetes Mellitus. Clinical Diabetes.
12. Shannon MH, Wintfeld N, Liang M, Jovanovic L. Pregnancy snapshot: a retrospective, observational case-control study to evaluate the potential effects of maternal diabetes treatment during pregnancy on macrosomia. Curr Med Res Opin. 2016;32(7):1183-92. doi: 10.1185/03007995.2016.1164128. Epub 2016 Apr 15.PubMed PMID: 26958899.

CHAPTER

19

Approach to a Child with Rickets

Anu Vishwanath

CASE

An 8-year-old male presents with concern for bilateral genu valgum deformity and complaint of pain in both lower limbs on walking or running. Parents note that he has always been the shortest boy in his class at school and his complaints of pain on walking and lower limb deformity have developed and progressed over the past six months. Patient and parents deny any trauma, and there is no history of fractures. Patient does not have any alopecia, or dental problems such as discoloration or abscesses. Patient has a history of polyuria and primary nocturnal enuresis.

Past Medical History

Patient has previously been healthy and there is no history of any prolonged illnesses or medications.

Birth History

Patient was born at full term by normal vaginal delivery. His birth weight was 3 kg and birth length was 48 cm. He had no discernable deformities at birth.

Diet History

Parents report that the patient consumes about 1500 kcal/day. Patient consumes dairy products including about 1–2 glasses of milk a day and about half to one cup of curd a day.

Family History

No family history of frequent fractures, bony deformities, dental problems or alopecia.

Social History

Patient lives at home with his parents and has an older sister who is reportedly healthy. Patient is in the 3rd standard and is doing well at school.

Physical Examination

Anthropometry

Weight 15 kg (–2.24 SD below mean weight for age), height 103 cm (–3.8 SD below mean height for age).

Head Circumference

50 cm, body mass index (BMI) 14.1 kg/m^2, body surface area (BSA) –0.65 m^2.

Vital Signs

Temperature: 36°C (axillary), pulse: 74/minute, respiratory rate: 14 breaths/min BP: 100/70 (right brachial, sitting position).

Patient appears small for his age, is conscious, oriented and interactive and complains of pain in his limbs. He has thin, lustureless, dull hair. There is widening at both his wrists. Patient has tenderness and widening over bilateral knee joints and there is bilateral genu valgum deformity. Abdomen appears slightly distended but no organomegaly is appreciated. Dental examination appears appropriate for his age, with no evidence of any dental caries or discoloration.

Evaluation

Patient is noted to have normal age appropriate serum calcium and phosphorus levels with elevated alkaline phosphatase of 547 U/L (145–420 U/L). 25 hydroxy vitamin D level is 14.33 ng/mL. 1,25 dihydroxy vitamin D level is elevated and PTH level is also elevated. He has normal blood glucose, urea and creatinine levels. His electrolyte panel shows serum sodium of 136 mEq/L, serum potassium 3.6 mEq/L, serum chloride of 107.5 mEq/L. Blood gas shows a bicarbonate of 15.1 mmol/L. Urine studies shows urine pH of 8.0, spot urine calcium/creatinine ratio is 0.805. His liver function tests, serum TSH are within age appropriate normal limits. Imaging studies shows bony changes consistent with rickets, and ultrasound of kidney evidence of nephrocalcinosis.

Q. 1 What are the etiologies of rickets?

- Rickets is characterized by deficient mineralization of bone osteoid at the growth plate in children.
- Osteomalacia refers to mineralization defects occurring after fusion of epiphyses.

Ans. Deficiency of vitamin D or genetic defects in action of vitamin D, calcium deficiency, phosphorus deficiency or phosphorus wasting, and renal tubular acidosis.

Etiologies—Rickets

- *Vitamin D Disorders:*
  - Vitamin D deficiency—nutritional deficiency, secondary to malabsorption, drugs,
  - Metabolic—Decreased liver 25-hydroxylase, vitamin D–dependent rickets type 1, vitamin D–dependent rickets type 2, renal or hepatic dysfunction
- *Calcium Deficiency:*
  - Nutritional deficiency, rickets of prematurity, malabsorption, increased loss in urine
- *Phosphorus Deficiency:*
  - Inadequate intake, rickets of prematurity, impaired absorption—such as due to aluminum-containing antacids
  - Increased urinary excretion of phosphorus
    - X-linked hypophosphatemic rickets, autosomal dominant hypophosphatemic rickets, autosomal recessive hypophosphatemic rickets, hereditary hypophosphatemic rickets with hypercalciuria
    - Overproduction of phosphatonins—tumor-induced osteomalacia, fibrous dysplasia (e.g. McCune-Albright syndrome), linear sebaceous nevus syndrome, neurofibromatosis
  - Renal tubular acidosis—Fanconi syndrome, Dent disease, cystinosis
- *Hypophosphatasia:*
  - Perinatal, infantile, childhood, adult onset

Q. 2 What are the features of rickets?

Ans.

- *Clinical features:*
  - *General features:* Failure to thrive, muscle weakness, fractures, increased susceptibility to infections
  - *Cranial and dental findings:* Craniotabes, delayed fontanelle closure, frontal bossing, delayed tooth eruption, poor enamel formation and caries, craniosynostosis
  - *Musculoskeletal findings:* Rachitic rosary–prominence of costochondral junctions, Harrison groove–indentation of the lower anterior thoracic wall with flaring of lower rib cage, pectus carinatum (chest wall deformity with anterior protrusion of sternum and adjacent costal cartilages), scoliosis (lateral curvature of spine), kyphosis (exaggerated thoracic spinal convexity posteriorly), lordosis (exaggerated lumbar spinal convexity anteriorly), enlargement of wrists and ankles, valgus or varus deformities predominantly noted at knees as either lateral bowing of legs or knock knee deformities, limb pain, anterior bowing of the tibia and femur.

- *Hypocalcemia symptoms:* Tetany, seizures, stridor due to laryngeal spasm

In children younger than 6 years, genu valgum deformity could be physiologic and self-limiting.

- *Radiologic features:* Osteopenia–lucency of bones, cupping, splaying, fraying of long bone metaphyses, widening of the physis
- *Histologic features:* Disorganized chondrocyte maturation, widened osteoid seams, undermineralization of trabeculae.

Q. 3 What investigations would be indicated in a case of rickets?

Ans.

- *Radiologic investigations:* X-ray with PA views of the wrist, knees, chest, ultrasound of kidney to assess for any nephrocalcinosis
- *Lab investigations:* Serum calcium, phosphorus, alkaline phosphatase, 25-hydroxy Vitamin D, PTH, 1,25-dihydroxy vitamin D, sodium, potassium, chloride, bicarbonate, anion gap, renal function (urea, creatinine)
  - Urine—pH, urine calcium, urine creatinine, urine glucose, urine protein, urinary phosphorus.

Q. 4 What is the trend of urinary calcium creatinine ratio with age?

Ans.

Age	Ca^{2+}/Cr ratio (mg/mg) (95th percentile for age)
<7 months	0.86
7–18 months	0.60
19 months–6 years	0.42
Adults	0.22

Q. 5 Who are at risk for developing nutritional vitamin D deficiency?

Ans. Dark-skinned individuals, premature infants, exclusively breastfed infants of mothers who are vitamin D deficient, individuals with limited exposure to sunlight, people residing at higher latitudes, diseases which lead to malabsorption of vitamin D such as celiac disease, biliary obstruction, pancreatic insufficiency, individuals on medications such as anticonvulsants.

Normal vitamin D levels
- Sufficiency—25 hydroxy vitamin D of 30–100 ng/mL
- Insufficiency—25 hydroxy vitamin D of 21–29 ng/mL
- Deficiency—25 hydroxy vitamin D below 20 ng/mL

Q. 6 How do you treat vitamin D deficiency in children?

Ans. To achieve a blood level of 25(OH)D above 30 ng/mL

- 1000 IU/day of vitamin D for about 6 weeks for infants less than 1 month old
- For children aged 1–18 years 2000 IU/day of vitamin D_2 (ergocalciferol) or Vitamin D_3 (cholecalciferol) for 6 weeks, or

With therapy, radiologic evidence of healing rickets is usually evident in 2–4 weeks in nutritional rickets.

- *Stoss therapy:* 100,000–600,000 IU of vitamin D orally (over 1–5 days) or 50,000 IU of vitamin once weekly for 6 weeks followed by maintenance therapy of 400–1000 IU/day (0–1 years) maintenance therapy of 600–1000 IU/day

Some patients with low calcium levels may also require supplementation with

- Calcium: 30–75 mg/kg/day of elemental calcium in 3 divided doses at the start of vitamin D therapy (doses to be weaned over 2–4 weeks)
- Calcitriol in doses of 20–100 ng/kg/day in 2–3 divided doses until calcium levels normalize.

Goals of treatment in rickets are to
- Relieve symptoms of pain
- Correct bony deformities
- Decrease the necessity for surgeries
- Improvement in growth
- Correct any underlying metabolic abnormality.

Q. 7 What forms of rickets do not respond to treatment with vitamin D?

Ans. Vitamin D dependent rickets type I (VDDR I) also known as VDDR IA or pseudovitamin D deficiency ricket type 1 (PDDR) is due to defective 1α-OHase (CYP27B1) activity leading to deficiency of biologically active form of vitamin D-calcitriol. The treatment usually is calcitriol 10–20 ng/kg/day in a single or two divided doses.

Another rare condition is a defect in vitamin D 25-hydroxylation due to mutation in the *CYP2R1* gene (also termed vitamin D-dependent rickets type 1B (VDDR IB).

Vitamin D-dependent rickets type II (VDDR II) also variably termed VDDR IIA or hereditary vitamin D-resistant rickets (HVDRR) which is due to resistance to the activated form of vitamin D, (calcitriol), usually manifests with rickets and features of alopecia and is associated with very high levels of calcitriol. The genetic defect is at the level of vitamin D receptor (*VDR*).

The VDDR IIB is due to an abnormal nuclear ribonucleoprotein that interferes with the vitamin D receptor-DNA interaction, leading to a phenotype similar to VDDR IIA with end-organ resistance to active vitamin D but a normal vitamin D receptor.

Management usually consists of high doses of calcitriol 1–6 μg/kg/day with supplemental calcium 1–3 g elemental daily, with the aim to achieve normocalcemia, to maintain PTH levels within normal limits and to avoid hypercalciuria. Some patients may require intravenous calcium supplementation 0.4–1.4 g elemental calcium/m^2/day to normalize calcium. Some patients with this form of rickets may spontaneously outgrow the defect as they enter puberty.

Other forms of rickets such as hypophosphatemic rickets or other causes listed previously need to be considered when a patient with rickets does not respond to vitamin D therapy.

Normal phosphorus levels in children
- 0–5 days—4.8–8.2 mg/dL
- 1–3 year—3.8–6.5 mg/dL
- 4–11 years—3.7–5.6 mg/dl
- 12–15 year—2.9–5.4 mg/dL
- 16–19 year—2.7–4.7 mg/dL

Q. 8 Describe the pathophysiology of hypophosphatemic rickets.

Ans. The main pathology is hypophosphatemia either due to dietary phosphate deficiency or due to renal phosphate wasting due to elevated phosphatonins which could be due to inherited genetic defects, or acquired due to tumors or medications.

Q. 9 Name some inherited disorders leading to hypophosphatemia.

Ans.

- X-linked hypophosphatemia (XLH) is an X-linked dominant disorder caused by loss of function of the phosphate-regulating gene with homology to endopeptidases located on the X-chromosome (*PHEX*), associated with elevation of FGF23.
- Autosomal recessive forms of hypophosphatemic rickets are caused by inactivating mutations in dentin matrix protein 1 (DMP1) and ectonucleotide pyrophosphatase/phosphodiesterase1 (*ENPP1*), also associated with excess fibroblast growth factor 23 (FGF23).
- Autosomal dominant hypophosphatemic rickets (ADHR) due to mutations in *FGF23* gene.

Q. 10 What are the clinical manifestations of hypophosphatemic rickets?

Ans. X-linked hypophosphatemia (XLH) may present in childhood with rickets and bone deformities, or in adulthood with muscle weakness, bone pain, fractures. Dental abscesses and enthesopathy (due to calcification of tendons and ligaments) may also be present.

ADHR usually has incomplete penetrance and has variable age of onset.

Q. 11 What is the approach to treatment of hypophosphatemic rickets?

Ans. Activated vitamin D calcitriol dosage of 20–30 ng/kg/day in 2–3 divided doses and an elemental phosphorus dose of 20–40 mg/kg/day (in 3–5 divided doses). Higher doses may be required at treatment initiation with periodic follow-up and dose titration.

Patient needs to be monitored for nephrocalcinosis, hypercalciuria, and hyperparathyroidism.

Q. 12 What are the important characters of renal tubular acidosis (RTA) and the diagnostic modalities?

Ans. Disorders of renal tubular acidification are due to defects in the reabsorption of bicarbonate (HCO_3^-), the excretion of hydrogen ion (H^+), or both. All types of RTA present with a normal anion gap (hyperchloremic) metabolic acidosis.

They are broadly classified as:

- Proximal RTA or type 2
- Distal RTA or type 1
- Combined proximal and distal RTA or type 3
- Hyperkalemic RTA or type 4.

The etiologies of RTA could be varied and result from primary intrinsic renal tubular defects or acquired secondary to other pathologies or drugs.

The basic laboratory work-up in any case of suspected RTA would need to include.

- Serum electrolytes and serum bicarbonate, plasma anion gap [Na^+–(Cl^-+HCO_3^-)]
- Urinary pH, urinary calcium, urinary creatinine
- Ultrasonography of the kidney to rule out nephrocalcinosis or obstructive uropathy.

Based on these tests further advanced tests to assess renal tubular function may be required.

Osteitis fibrosa cystica, is the term used to describe the classic radiological manifestation of hyperparathyroidism.

- Generalized skeletal demineralization
- Subperiosteal bone resorption with cortical thinning
- Brown tumors (osteoclastomas)—lytic lesions and bone cysts that can disrupt the overlying cortex
- Salt and pepper appearance on skull radiographs

Q. 13 What is the management of RTA?

Ans.

Any underlying disease leading to RTA has to be identified and managed. Patients with proximal RTA require bicarbonate equivalent up to 20 mEq/kg/day in the form of sodium bicarbonate or sodium citrate solution.

Patients with distal RTAs generally require 2–4 mEq/kg/day bicarbonate equivalent and should be monitored for the development of hypercalciuria. Those with symptomatic hypercalciuria, nephrocalcinosis, or nephrolithiasis (recurrent episodes of gross hematuria) may require thiazide diuretics to decrease urine calcium excretion.

Electrolyte abnormalities such as hypokalemia, hyperkalemia and hypophosphatemia need to be monitored with appropriate therapy.

Q. 14 Describe the pathophysiology and management in renal rickets.

Ans. Many of the disorders leading to hypophosphatemia and renal tubular acidosis involve renal tubular defects.

An other form of metabolic bone disease is associated with chronic kidney disease (CKD), previously termed renal osteodystrophy. Bone abnormalities in CKD include:

- High bone turnover disease related to secondary hyperparathyroidism
- Low turnover disease or adynamic bone disease.

The hyperphosphatemia, uremia and acidosis due to CKD leads to a cascade of events leading to deficiency of calcitriol and secondary hyperparathyroidism.

Treatment involves administration of activated form of vitamin D (calcitriol) 0.01–0.05 μg/kg/day, dietary phosphorus restriction and use of phosphorus binders to decrease absorption of phosphorus, correction of acidosis.

Follow-up of clinical case: Based on the finding of low serum bicarbonate with elevated urinary pH, with nephrocalcinosis, a diagnosis of distal renal tubular acidosis is made. Patient is started on sodium citrate solution, to treat the metabolic acidosis with close follow-up growth and bone deformities.

SUGGESTED READING

1. Agarwal DK, et al. Physical and sexual growth pattern of affluent Indian children from 5 to 18 years of age. Indian Pediatrics. 1992.
2. Carpenter TO, Imel EA, Holm IA, Jan de Beur SM, Insogna KL. A clinician's guide to X-linked hypophosphatemia. J Bone Miner Res. 2011;26(7):1381-8. doi: 10.1002/jbmr.340. Epub 2011 May 2.
3. Holick MF, Binkley NC, Bischoff-Ferrari HA, Gordon CM, Hanley DA, Heaney RP, et al. Evaluation, treatment, and prevention of vitamin D deficiency: an Endocrine Society clinical practice guideline; Endocrine society. J Clin Endocrinol Metab. 2011;96(7):1911-30. doi:10.1210/jc. 2011-0385. Epub 2011 jun 6.
4. Imel EA1, Econs MJ. Approach to the hypophosphatemic patient. J Clin Endocrinol Metab; 2012.
5. Linglart A1, Biosse-Duplan M, Briot K, Chaussain C, Esterle L, Guillaume-Czitrom S, et al. Therapeutic management of hypophosphatemic rickets from infancy to adulthood. Endocr Connect. 2014;3(1):R13-30. doi: 10.1530/EC-13-0103. Print 2014.
6. Meites S (Ed). Pediatric Clinical Chemistry, 3rd edn. Washington, DC: American Association for Clinical Chemistry, 1989.
7. Misra M, Pacaud D, Petryk A, Collett Solberg PF, Kappy M; Drug and therapeutic committee of the Lawson wilking Pediatric Endocrine Society; Endocrine society. Vitamin D deficiency in children and its management: review of current knowledge and recommendations. Pediatrics. 2008;122(2):398-417. doi:10.1542/peds. 2007-1894.
8. Sargent JD, Stukel TA, Kresel J, et al. Normal values for random urinary calcium to creatinine ratios in infancy. J Pediatr. 1993.

Index

Page numbers followed by *b* refer to box, *f* refer to figure, *fc* refer to flowchart, and *t* refer to table.

A

B

C

D

E

F

G

H

P

R

S

T

U

V

W